Instructor's Manual

for
Swanson and Nies

Community Health Nursing: Promoting the Health of Aggregates

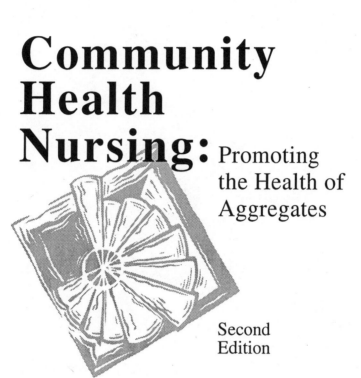

Second Edition

Melanie McEwen, PhD, RN, CS
Associate Professor
Baylor University School of Nursing
Dallas, Texas

A printed testbank is available from the publisher to all adopters.

W.B. SAUNDERS COMPANY
A Division of Harcourt Brace & Company

Philadelphia London Toronto
Montreal Sydney Tokyo

W.B. SAUNDERS COMPANY

A Division of Harcourt Brace & Company

The Curtis Center
Independence Square West
Philadelphia, Pennsylvania 19106-3399

Icons by Lingta Kung.

Instructor's Manual for Swanson and Nies
COMMUNITY HEALTH NURSING:
Promoting the Health of Aggregates, second edition   ISBN 0–7216–6168–8

Printed in the United States of America.

Last digit is the print number: 9 8 7 6 5 4 3 2 1

CONTENTS

INTRODUCTION

This manual was written to assist instructors in preparing lectures and planning learning experiences related to the content of *Community Health Nursing: Promoting the Health of Aggregates* (2nd edition). The manual is arranged in chapters that correspond to the chapters in the textbook. Each manual chapter is divided into three sections: Annotated Learning Objectives, Chapter Outline, and Teaching Strategies. In addition, a rate calculations worksheet, a community assessment tool, and overhead transparency masters of chapter heading outlines, figures, and tables are provided. A separate Test Manual contains chapter examination questions.

The Annotated Learning Objectives section briefly answers each objective. The purpose of this section is to present the material in a concise, understandable format that will allow the instructor to draw out quickly important points in lecture preparation. The annotated learning objectives might also be used as an answer key, should the instructor choose to design an essay examination based on the learning objectives.

The Lecture Outline section summarizes the major concepts and content of each chapter. It is designed to be used as an aid to organize the material for presentation. Appendix B contains heading outlines for each chapter to be used to create transparencies for use during lecture. Tables, figures, illustrations, and graphs contained in the book have also been enlarged and included in the manual to create transparencies for use during lectures to promote discussion and enhance explanation for some of the key points.

The Teaching Strategies section contains suggestions instructors can add to their repertory of classroom skills and techniques. In many cases, the use of guest speakers is encouraged to expand on the material presented in the text and allow the students to listen to, talk to, and learn from nurses who participate in various types of aggregate practice. Other teaching strategies include a variety of exercises to encourage application and understanding of the material. Community and family assessments, calculation of morbidity and mortality rates, field trips and group discussions are examples of approaches suggested.

This manual is designed to provide a foundation to facilitate lecture and discussion preparation for the community health nursing instructor. It is also hoped that the manual will promote presentation of the material in a manner that makes nursing care of aggregates appealing to students and encourages community health nursing as a potential career choice.

Health: A Community View

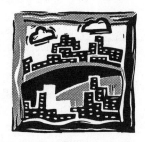

ANNOTATED LEARNING OBJECTIVES

1. Compare and contrast definitions of health as used in public health nursing.

The definition of health is evolving. Health can be defined in social terms, as seen in the classic definition by the World Health Organization (WHO): "a state of complete physical, mental, and social well-being and not merely the absence of disease or infirmity."

Health can also be seen as a continuum, with illness and peak wellness at the extremes. It is typically defined in terms of the individual. From the community/public health perspective, however, health is defined in relation to individuals, families, groups, and communities.

Health is also relative. Nurses working in the community should understand how the community defines its own health. When working in a particular community, nurses should obtain definitions from families, organizations, and aggregates in that community.

2. Define and discuss the focus of public health.

According to Winslow, "Public health is the science and art of preventing disease, prolonging life, and promoting health and efficiency through organized community effort. . . ." Public health connotes efforts made through public channels such as government agencies (health departments), which serve the people in accordance with legislation and are supported by taxes. Its focus is to promote and preserve the health of populations. Public health policy directs lifestyle changes as well as social and environmental changes.

Public health is based on the principle of social justice, which entitles everyone to basic necessities such as adequate income and health care. Unlike the predominant U.S. model of market justice, which entitles people to only what they have gained through individual efforts, public health accepts collective burdens to provide basic services for all.

3. List the three levels of prevention and give one example of each.

Disease prevention activities protect people from disease and its consequences. The three levels of prevention that are widely recognized in public health are:

Primary prevention—activities that prevent a problem before it occurs. MMR and DPT immunizations are examples of primary prevention.

Secondary prevention—activities that provide early detection and intervention. Screening such as mammography, blood pressure checks, and glaucoma tests are examples of secondary prevention.

Tertiary prevention—activities that correct a disease state and prevent further deterioration. Examples of tertiary prevention include providing physical therapy following CVA and teaching a newly diagnosed diabetic how to perform insulin injections.

4. Differentiate between the conceptual models of community health nursing as defined by the American Nurses' Association and of public health nursing as defined by the American Public Health Association.

Community health nursing—According to the ANA, "community health nursing is a synthesis of nursing practice and public health practice applied to promoting and preserving the health of populations." Practice is continual, not episodic. It is general and comprehensive; its chief responsibility is the population as a whole.

Public health nursing (PHN)—The APHA defines public health nursing as nursing that "synthesizes the body of knowledge from the public health sciences and professional nursing theories for the purpose of improving the health of the entire community." The goals of PHN are primary prevention and health promotion.

Comparison—Both definitions address the provision of nursing service to meet health needs of aggregates or the community. Both definitions combine concepts and practices from public health and nursing.

Contrast—The ANA definition focuses on care to individuals, families, and groups within a community. Community health nursing practice involves working with smaller groups to correct community problems.

The APHA definition focuses on care to the community as a whole. It considers the individual or family only as a member of a group at risk.

LECTURE OUTLINE

I. **Introduction: Characteristics of the U.S. Health Care System**
    A. In the United States, health care is moving from a disease-oriented system to one that is health-oriented. Health care costs increased from 5.9% of the gross domestic product in 1965 to 13.9% in 1993, with expenditures exceeding $3299 per person. Currently, hospital care makes up 37% of health care costs, and physician services account for 19%, but preventive public health activities account for only 3% of health care costs.
    B. Nurses are the largest group of health care providers. In 1992, about 66.5% of employed RNs worked in hospitals, and about 15% worked in community, school, or occupational health settings. However, it is predicted that there will be a marked decline in hospital employment of nurses and an increase in the number of nurses working in community settings that focus on health promotion and preventive care.

II. **Definitions of Health**
    A. The World Health Organization defines health as "a state of complete physical, mental, and social well-being and not merely the absence of disease or infirmity."
    B. Several other definitions of health focus chiefly on the individual. Most definitions include complex concepts such as stress, adaptation, environment, goals, fluidity, and wellness.

C. In community health nursing practice, it is important to understand how the community and various aggregates within it define health.

III. **Definitions of Public Health and Community Health**
    A. "Public health is the science and art of
       1. Preventing disease
       2. Prolonging life and
       3. Promoting health and efficiency through organized community effort . . ." (Winslow)
    B. The term *public health* includes the efforts of government agencies that are supported by taxes and run in accordance with legislation.
       1. Public health services are provided at the federal, state, and local levels.
       2. Federal and state services are mainly supportive and advisory, whereas local levels provide direct services to the public.
       3. Services provided at the local levels include efforts to protect the public through sanitation; air and water pollution control; and personal health care services such as immunization, family planning, and care for people with STDs. Public health efforts are multidisciplinary.

IV. **Preventive Approach to Health**
    A. Health promotion and levels of prevention
       1. *Health promotion* enhances resources aimed at improving well-being.
       2. *Disease prevention* protects people from disease and its consequences. There are three levels of prevention.
          a. *Primary prevention* prevents a problem before it occurs.
          b. *Secondary prevention* provides early detection and intervention.
          c. *Tertiary prevention* corrects a disease state and prevents it from causing further deterioration.
    B. Prevention versus cure: Can we afford one over the other?
       1. Spending money on "cure" does not improve the health of the population. Prevention, however, does.
       2. The real determinants of health are prevention efforts such as education, housing, food, a decent income, and a safe social and physical environment.
       3. Continual overexpansion of health care may harm the health of the population by diverting a disproportionate part of expenditures away from other necessities such as schools, roads, housing, and food.

V. **Public and Community Health Nursing**
  A. APHA definition
    1. "Public health nursing synthesizes the body of knowledge from the public health sciences and professional nursing theories for the purpose of improving the health of the entire community."
    2. Primary prevention and health promotion provide the basis for public health nursing practice.
    3. The focus of public health nursing is on care to the community as a whole; individuals and families are viewed as members of groups at risk.
  B. ANA definition
    1. "Community health nursing is a synthesis of nursing practice and public health practice applied to promoting and preserving the health of populations."
    2. Community health nursing is general, comprehensive, and continuing, with nursing care directed to individuals, families, or groups to promote the health of the total population.
    3. "Health promotion, health maintenance, health education and management, coordination, and continuity of care are utilized."
  C. Community/Public Health Advanced Practice Nursing (C/PHAPN)
    1. C/PHAPN is a type of clinical nursing specialization in which the nurse functions in administrative and clinical roles focusing on populations or communities.
    2. Practice includes promotion, maintenance, protection, and restoration of health, as well as prevention of disease and disability for communities, aggregates, and other groups of individuals who share common characteristics.
    3. A minimum of a master's degree is required for C/PHAPN.
  D. Population-focused practice
    1. Community health nurses do not simply provide direct care to individuals and families. Instead, they use a population-focused approach.
    2. Population-focused care is based on a community assessment process that leads to planning, intervention, and evaluation at the individual, family, aggregate, and population levels.
    3. Population-focused practice is concerned with many subpopulations within the community.
    4. Data collection is ongoing, not episodic.
    5. Preparation for community health nursing
      a. A *Generalist Community Health Nurse* has a baccalaureate degree. Nurses with this degree plan and intervene with individuals, groups, aggregates, and subpopulations.
      b. A *Specialist Community Health Nurse* has graduate preparation. Nurses with this degree plan and intervene with multiple and overlapping subpopulations within a community.
  E. Aggregate-focused practice
    1. Community health nurses focus on aggregates in settings such as homes, clinics, and schools.
    2. They must be able to assess the aggregate's health needs and resources, identify its values and value systems, and work with the community to identify and implement programs to meet health needs and evaluate program effectiveness.

VI. **Managed Care**
  A. The term *managed care* typically refers to the organization and management of health care for an enrolled group of individuals. The individuals belonging to the health care organization may be viewed as the population served.
  B. Managed care organizations are similar to public health agencies in that both seek to improve health within their populations. To accomplish this, managed care organizations use many strategies, such as promoting healthy lifestyles, providing preventive and primary care, expanding and ensuring access to cost-effective and technologically appropriate care, participating in coordinated and interdisciplinary care, and involving patients and families in decision-making.

TEACHING STRATEGIES

1. Provide students with complete ANA and APHA definitions of community and public health nursing. Form student groups, and have the groups compare and contrast these definitions.
2. Have students brainstorm to list activities and services performed by community health nurses. Have students classify each as health promotion or primary, secondary, or tertiary prevention. Discuss the possibilities for overlap among these categories.
3. Invite a C/PHAPN to speak to the class about the role of the specialist in community health nursing.

Historical Factors: Community Health Nursing in Context

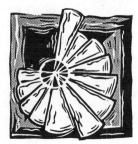

ANNOTATED LEARNING OBJECTIVES

1. **Describe the impact of the aggregate on the health of populations from the hunting and gathering stage to the present.**

   Increased population, adaptation to the environment, and lifestyle changes have affected aggregate health throughout the centuries. During the hunting and gathering stage, nutrition was probably good, infectious diseases were rare, and waste disposal was not a problem. However, individuals probably suffered from a variety of problems such as parasites and insect bites. During the settled village stage, the number of diseases passed from animals to humans increased, nutrient deficiencies were common, and inadequate clean water and waste disposal were beginning to become problems. In the preindustrial cities stage, the problems with clean water and waste disposal worsened, and diseases related to these problems developed. Increases in other communicable diseases also occurred. During the industrial cities stage, air and water pollution were severe, and working conditions were harsh. Infectious diseases were numerous, and many epidemics and pandemics occurred. Diseases in the present stage often result from sedentary lifestyles, poor personal habits and environmental hazards and stressors. Although food is abundant, diets are frequently unhealthy.

2. **Trace approaches to the health of aggregates from prehistoric times to the present.**

   In *prehistoric times,* efforts to manage health included psychosomatic medicine, isolation, and fumigation. During *Classical times,* drainage systems were built, pharmaceutical preparations were employed, methods and rules for cleanliness and management of communicable disease were used, and embalming the dead was practiced. In the *Middle Ages,* primary health care was provided by religious leaders who applied religion and magic to health problems. Public health measures included controlling the water supply and refuse disposal. Communicable diseases were rampant. During the *Renaissance,* communicable diseases spread as a result of population growth and migration. Efforts to care for the poor were begun, and microscopic organisms were discovered. In the *18th and 19th centuries,* problems with sanitation increased, and communicable diseases flourished. Child labor was also an increasing problem. Vaccination against smallpox was begun. The Chadwick Report (Great Britain, 1842) and the Shattuck Report (Massachusetts, 1850) described health conditions and made recommendations for public health reform.

3. **Analyze three historical events that have influenced a holistic approach to the health of populations.**

   The *germ theory of disease* was proposed by Pasteur in 1854. Discoveries of the cause of tuberculosis and cholera (Koch) and rabies (Pasteur), as well as the successful use of antiseptics by Lister, supported the germ theory. These events encouraged a focus on the individual organism as the cause of disease. As a result, diagnosis and treatment(s) were organism- or disease-specific.

   The *Flexner Report* (1910) brought about profound changes in medical education in the United States, emphasizing the utilization of scientific theory in medicine. Again, the single agent (germ) theory of illness was supported, and focus centered on disease and symptoms.

   The *Johns Hopkins School of Public Health* was established in 1916 by the Rockefeller Foundation. It focused on the preservation and improvement of individual and community health and on disease prevention.

4. Compare the application of the principles of public health to the nation's major health problem at the turn of the century (infectious disease) with that in the 1990s (chronic illness).

In the early 1900s, public health efforts such as improved nutrition, increased food production, water purification, sewage disposal, improved food handling and pasteurization of milk contributed greatly to the decrease in communicable illnesses which were common at that time. In contrast, chronic illness is the major health problem of the 1990s. Public health efforts therefore must begin to focus on healthful living (Hygeia) as opposed to finding a cure (Panacea). Multicausal views of disease, which consider environment, stress and lifestyle factors, are needed to explain the major health problems of the late 20th century.

5. Describe two leaders in nursing who had a profound impact on addressing the health of aggregates.

Florence Nightingale—Her work concentrated on the influence of environmental factors on health. She emphasized sanitation and community assessment and analysis. She was also a renowned statistician and advocated the use of statistics to direct health interventions.

Lillian Wald—With Mary Brewster, Wald began Henry Street House in New York. She was also instrumental in beginning school nursing and worked with Metropolitan Life to use health education and health promotion to decrease morbidity and mortality. She was a founder and the first president of the Association of Public Health Nurses.

6. Discuss two major contemporary issues facing community health nursing, and trace their historical roots to the present.

Although there have been changes over the centuries, problems with environmental pollution, particularly of air and water, caused by industrialization are still with us. Communicable disease outbreaks and epidemics such as AIDS, STDs, influenza and tuberculosis can be traced to lifestyles, living conditions, availability of health information and health care, and other factors.

Infant and maternal morbidity and mortality have improved dramatically over the years; however, they are still significantly higher than necessary. Lack of adequate, accessible, affordable health care for many aggregates contributes to these problems.

LECTURE OUTLINE

I. **Evolution of the State of Health of Western Populations**—Increasing population and popula-

tion density have resulted in environmental changes that have caused ecological imbalance. These changes have had a progressive impact on the state of health in Western populations.

A. Hunting and gathering stage
 1. Populations consisted of small groups that wandered in search of foods.
 2. Nutrition was probably good due to the availability of a variety of nutrients.
 3. People probably suffered from parasites (lice and pinworms), insect bites, and related illnesses.
 4. There were few contagious diseases because of lack of interaction.
 5. Waste disposal was not a problem.
B. Settled village stage
 1. Small groups of people settled together in permanent dwellings.
 2. Zoonoses (diseases capable of being passed from animals to humans), nutrient deficiencies, and problems related to agrarian lifestyles increased.
 3. Waste disposal and water availability were becoming problems.
C. Preindustrial cities stage
 1. Waste disposal and the availability of a clean water supply became increasing problems. As a result, diseases such as cholera and plague were common.
 2. The incidence of other communicable diseases also increased.
D. Industrial cities stage
 1. Industrialization produced large amounts of waste that resulted in heavy air and water pollution and harsh working conditions.
 2. Epidemics of infectious diseases such as tuberculosis, diphtheria, smallpox and measles proliferated.
E. Present stage
 1. Sedentary lifestyles and negative personal behaviors (smoking, substance abuse) have an adverse effect on health.
 2. Dietary changes and individual behaviors have produced an increase in bowel diseases, venous disorders, and heart disease.
 3. An increase in some communicable diseases, associated with overcrowding, can also be seen.

II. **Evolution of Early Public Health Efforts**
A. Prehistoric times—Crude efforts were taken to manage health, including psychosomatic medicine (voodoo), isolation (banishment) and fumigation (smoke).
B. Classical times (3000–1400 B.C.)

1. Drainage systems were built, methods to embalm the dead were instituted, and pharmaceutical preparations were developed.
2. The *Mosaic Law* prescribed rules for cleanliness and management of communicable disease.

C. Middle Ages
1. Priests and monks became the primary health care providers, and they applied both religion and magic to health problems.
2. Communicable diseases such as diphtheria, smallpox, leprosy and bubonic plague were rampant and, in some cases, pandemic.
3. Public health measures included building wells and fountains, cleaning the streets, and disposing of refuse.

D. Renaissance (14th-15th centuries)
1. Population growth and migration characterized this period.
2. *Von Leeuwenhoek* discovered microscopic organisms.
3. The *Elizabethan Poor Law* (1601) placed care for the poor under the guidance of the local parishes.

E. Eighteenth century
1. Imperialism and industrialization produced many problems with sanitation.
2. Poor children were forced into labor.
3. *Jenner* began vaccinating against smallpox.

F. Nineteenth century
1. Unsanitary conditions remained.
2. Communicable diseases such as typhus and typhoid fever killed thousands.
3. The *Chadwick Report* (1842) described health conditions and life expectancy of the poor in Great Britain and resulted in the establishment of the General Board of Health for England.

III. **Advent of Modern Health Care**
A. Florence Nightingale and the evolution of modern nursing
1. Modern nursing began in the mid-1800s largely through the efforts of Florence Nightingale.
2. Much of her work centered on the influence of environmental factors on health. She emphasized sanitation, community assessment and analysis, the use of statistics and the gathering of census data, and political advocacy on the behalf of aggregates.
3. In addition to her valuable work in nursing, her contributions with regard to the application of statistics to health and health care were vitally important.

B. Establishment of modern medical care and public health practice
1. Prior to 1900, physicians were trained in apprenticeships. Treatments included bloodletting, leeches, and administration of doses of metals. Iatrogenic diseases were rampant.
2. Several discoveries led to the acceptance of the germ theory of disease (proposed by Pasteur in 1854) and encouraged a focus on the individual organism and the individual disease in diagnosis and treatment.
   a. Pasteur proposed the germ theory in 1854.
   b. Koch discovered the cause of tuberculosis and cholera.
   c. Lister began using antiseptics for surgical supplies.
   d. Pasteur discovered rabies vaccination (1885) and determined the cause of puerperal fever.
3. Allopathism (treatment of the part) rather than holism (considering the social, economic, and environmental context as a whole contributing to a disease) influenced the direction of medical care and public health.
4. Social reforms to contain the spread of contagions led to the formation of local boards of health to safeguard water and food, manage sewage, and quarantine contagious disease victims.
5. The Johns Hopkins Medical School was established in 1885.
6. The Flexner Report (1910) brought about profound changes in medical education by closing "inadequate" schools and emphasizing the use of scientific theory in medicine. Consequences included a focus on the "single agent theory" of illness and on disease and symptoms rather than on therapy, prevention of disability, and holism.
7. The Johns Hopkins School of Public Health was begun in 1916 by the Rockefeller Foundation. Its focus was on the preservation and improvement of health in individuals and the community and the prevention of disease through multidisciplinary efforts.

IV. **Community Caregiver**
A. The community caregiver is a traditional role still common in non-western cultures. The role of the "healer" is integrated with other social institutions such as religion, medicine, and morality.

B. Some aspects of modern nursing, in particular public health nursing, evolved from practice in the home and developed, in part, from the community caregiver role.

V. **Establishment of Public Health Nursing**
   A. Public health nursing developed from providing nursing care to the sick poor and helping the poor by providing information and advocacy.
   B. District nursing was developed in England and endorsed by William Rathbone. District nurses and social workers were assigned to meet individual health needs and deliver nursing care and health education.
   C. Health visiting began in Manchester in 1862 to provide home visitors who would give health information to the poor. Health visiting was later combined with district nursing.
   D. Public health nursing in the United States began in the late 1800s.
      1. The first Visiting Nurses Associations were set up in Buffalo (1885) and Philadelphia (1886).
      2. Lillian Wald and Mary Brewster established a district nursing service called Henry Street House in New York (1893). Their philosophy was to meet the health needs of aggregates and to help people help themselves.
      3. Lillian Wald was also instrumental in beginning school nursing in New York (1902). Linda Rogers was the first school nurse.
      4. In 1912, the National Organization of Public Health Nursing was formed, and Lillian Wald was elected president.

VI. **Consequences for the Health of Aggregates**
   A. New causes for mortality—Death rates from infectious diseases declined in the 18th and 19th centuries. This decline was attributable to better nutrition, increased food production, water purification, sewage disposal, improved food handling and pasteurization of milk. Medicine and immunization programs had little effect until the 1920s and 1930s.
   B. Hygeia vs. Panacea—The debate over the relative importance of healthful living (Hygeia) vs. "cure" (Panacea) still exists. The focus of medical technology and academic sciences has stressed specific, disease-focused causation. A shift needs to be made to identify major determinants of health and prevention of disease and disability.
   C. Additional theories of disease causation—The germ theory is a unicausal model and is not sufficient to explain all disease.

VII. **Challenges for Community Health Nursing**
   A. Community health nurses must work to promote the health of populations.
   B. When planning interventions, nurses should consider the new causes of morbidity and mortality.
   C. Nurses should be encouraged to focus on underserved populations and the provision of holistic care.
   D. Education in community health nursing is greatly needed.

TEACHING STRATEGIES

1. Collect newspaper articles describing outbreaks of communicable diseases such as measles, cholera, or AIDS and discuss public health efforts to reduce or eliminate them. Also discuss personal habits, living conditions, and other factors that contribute to the spread of the disease.
2. Obtain 19th or early 20th century medical, nursing, or public health textbooks. Read and discuss exerpts with the class. What has changed? What has remained the same?

CHAPTER

3

The Health Care System

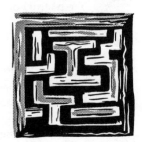

ANNOTATED LEARNING OBJECTIVES

1. **Describe the private health care subsystem and the public health subsystem.**

    The U.S. health care system is divided into two subsystems. The private health care subsystem focuses on the individual and is provided by for-profit and non-profit sectors and personal care physicians. This subsystem focuses on health promotion; early detection, diagnosis, and treatment of disease; and disease prevention. Services are provided in clinics, physicians' offices, homes, hospitals, and skilled care facilities.

    The public health care subsystem is concerned with the health of populations and the provision of a healthy environment. It is composed of federal, state, and local levels of government programs.

2. **Analyze landmark health care legislation and its impact on the delivery system.**

    The impact of federal legislation on the provision of health care is extensive. Numerous acts, programs, and agencies have influenced health care. Among them are the *Shepard-Towner Act* (1921), which provides funds for health and welfare of infants; the *Social Security Act* (1935, 1965, and 1972), which provides welfare for mothers and children and health care for the elderly and the handicapped; establishment of the *Department of Health, Education, and Welfare* (now Health and Human Services) in 1953; and the *Nurse Training Act* (1964), which provided funds for scholarships and training for nurses. In an effort to decrease federal spending, the Social Security Amendment of 1983 instituted a prospective payment system for Medicare with reimbursement based on diagnostic-related groups (DRGs).

3. **Describe the organization of the public health care subsystem at the national, state, and local levels.**

    Federal—The Department of Health and Human Services (DHHS) is the main organizational body of the public health care system at the federal level. DHHS is divided into five major agencies: Office of Human Development, Health Care Financing Administration, Social Security Administration, Family Support Administration, and the U.S. Public Health Service.

    State—At the state level, public health organization varies greatly, depending on the population and the geographic size of the state. Public health efforts may be directed by a board of health or may be overseen by a health officer. Nurses are the largest group of professionals at the state level.

    Local—At the local level, public health agencies are responsible for direct delivery of health care. As at the state level, organization varies greatly depending on the population and geographic size. Local efforts may be carried out at the city, municipality, county, or parish level.

4. **Describe the scope of the public health care subsystem at all levels.**

    Federal—The federal government focuses on the health of the general population, various special populations, and the international community. It also directs efforts to improve health habits, improve nutrition, and prevent substance abuse.

    State—The role of the state in public health varies greatly from state to state. Assessment of vital statistics, epidemiological activities, laboratory analyses, policy development, licensure, inspection, environmental safety activities, health education, and resource development are among the services offered.

Local—Local public health agencies determine the health status and needs of their constituents, identify unmet needs, and act to meet those needs. Services include environmental health services (safe water and food, pollution control, and sanitation); community health services (communicable disease surveillance, immunization); mental health services; and personal health services (care to individuals in clinics, schools, etc.).

5. *Describe the goals for health care in the future.*

Future goals for health care will depend on changing demographics and changing health problems. Chronic diseases (AIDS, heart disease, cancer), the aging of the population, escalating health care costs, increased technology, and environmental hazards all will have an impact on health care. Goals will increasingly focus on disease prevention and health promotion with recognition of, and intervention toward, social and behavioral factors that influence health. Health care for all will be provided by collaborative federal/state/local effort and by networking between private and public agencies.

LECTURE OUTLINE

I. **Major Legislation and the Health Care System**—Health care legislation generally involves either prevention of illness through influence on the environment or provision of funding to support programs that impact health care provision.
 A. Pure Food and Drugs Act (1906)—one of the first legislative attempts to prevent morbidity and mortality due to environmental influences
 B. Children's Bureau (1912)—protected children from unhealthy child labor practices
 C. Shepard-Towner Act (1921)—provided funds for health and welfare of infants
 D. Hill-Burton Act—provided federal funding for construction of hospitals
 E. Department of Health, Education, and Welfare—established in 1953 (became Health and Human Services in 1979)
 F. Nurse Training Act (1964)—provided funds for loans and scholarships for training nurses
 G. Social Security Act (1935, amended in 1965 and 1972)—provided welfare for mothers and children and health care for the elderly and handicapped; established Medicare and Medicaid
   1. Medicare—Title XVIII Social Security Amendment (1965)—is a federal program that pays specified health care services for all people over the age of 65 years and for eligible people with permanent total disabilities. It is funded through a payroll tax for all working citizens.
     a. Medicare Part A pays for hospital, nursing home, and skilled home health services. Part A has no monthly premium, but it requires copayments and places limitations on the type and duration of services available.
     b. Medicare Part B pays for physician, outpatient, home health, and ambulatory care. It requires a monthly fee and is voluntary.
     c. Medicare does not cover prescription drugs, preventive services, long-term care, or dental care.
   2. Medicaid—Title XIX Social Security Amendment (1965)— is a joint federal and state program that provides access to care for the poor and medically indigent of all ages. Federal funds are allocated to states on a matching basis (50% of costs are paid by the federal government). To be eligible for matching federal funds, states must offer basic services such as hospital care, physical therapy, laboratory, and home health care. States may also include optional services such as drugs, eyeglasses, inpatient psychiatric care, and dental care. Eligibility criteria are based on level of income and vary from state to state.
 H. National Health Planning and Resources Act (1974)—established "health service areas" and encouraged development of state and local health policy
 I. Omnibus Budget Reconciliation Act (1981)—reduced eligibility of poor women and children for welfare and health care
 J. Social Security Act Amendment (1983)—instituted a prospective payment system for Medicare with reimbursement being based on diagnostic-related groups (DRGs)
 K. Family Support Act (1988)—expanded coverage for poor women and children and extended Medicaid and AFDC
 L. Health Objectives Act 2000 (1990)—established health objectives for improvement of health status of United States citizens by the year 2000

II. **Redefining Health**
 A. Definition: "Health is a state characterized by anatomic integrity; ability to perform personally

valued family, work, and community roles; ability to deal with physical, biologic, and social stress; a feeling of well-being; and freedom from the risk of disease and untimely death." The focus of health care services is changing from illness care to promoting a safe environment, protecting health, promoting healthier lifestyles, improving nutrition, and providing health services.

  B. Determinants of health
   1. Four major inputs that determine health
    a. Heredity
    b. Health care services
    c. Behavior
    d. Environment
   2. Measurable outcomes of a health care system
    a. Life span
    b. Disease
    c. Discomfort
    d. Participation in health care
    e. Health behavior
    f. Social behavior
    g. Satisfaction
   3. Goals for the health care system
    a. Promotion of high-level "wellness"
    b. Promotion of satisfaction with the environment
    c. Minimization of departures from physiologic or functional norms for optimal health
    d. Prolongation of life through prevention of premature death
    e. Extension of resistance to ill health and creation of reserve capacity
    f. Minimization of illness
    g. Minimization of incapacity or disability
    h. Increase in capacity for underprivileged people to participate in health matters
  C. Prevention of disease and promotion of health—In the United States, health promotion is usually interpreted as modification of lifestyle to prevent disease (such as exercise, smoking cessation, good nutritional habits, and weight control).

III. **Components of the Health Care System**
  A. Private health care subsystem
   1. The private health care subsystem focuses on health promotion, prevention and early detection of disease, and diagnosis and treatment of disease.
   2. Care is focused on individuals by non-profit and for-profit sectors and by personal care physicians.

   3. The private subsystem focuses on cure, rehabilitative and restorative care, and custodial care of individuals.
   4. Services are provided on an outpatient basis in clinics, physicians' offices, hospital ambulatory centers, and homes, and on an inpatient basis in hospitals and skilled care facilities.
   5. Models of personal care (physician practice)
    a. Solo practice of a physician in an office
    b. Single-specialty group in which several physicians share resources and pool expenses
    c. Multi-specialty group practice that allows interaction across specialty areas
    d. Integrated health maintenance model staffed with prepaid multi-specialty physicians
    e. Community health centers that address issues such as education and housing and their impact on health
   6. Voluntary agencies—foundations set up by wealthy businesspeople to provide funds for charitable endeavors to meet health needs. They may be categorized according to their primary concern.
    a. Specific diseases (American Diabetes Association, American Cancer Society)
    b. Specific organ or body structure (National Kidney Foundation, American Heart Association)
    c. Health and welfare of a special group (National Council on Aging)
    d. Particular phase of health (Planned Parenthood)
    e. Professional organizations (American Nurses Association, American Medical Association)
  B. Public health care subsystem
   1. The public subsystem is concerned with the health of populations and the provision of a healthy environment. It includes efforts organized by society to protect, promote, and restore the people's health. It is mandated by law to address the health needs of populations.
   2. This subsystem is composed of programs at the federal, state, and local levels of government.
   3. Programs, services, and institutions involved emphasize the prevention of disease and the health needs of the population as a whole.

4. Roles of public health
   a. To search for causes of disease
   b. To develop ways to protect the public against disease
   c. To establish programs to address health problems

IV. **Roles of the Federal Government in Public Health**
   A. Organization—The Department of Health and Human Services (DHHS) implements and administers most activities. DHHS is composed of five major agencies.
      1. Office of Human Development Services is responsible for programs that meet special needs of the population.
      2. Health Care Financing Administration administers Medicare and Medicaid.
      3. Social Security Administration administers all services related to income for the aged, blind, and disabled.
      4. Family Support Administration works to strengthen the family unit.
      5. U.S. Public Health Service has six units.
         a. Centers for Disease Control (CDC) work to prevent and control infectious diseases and performs many other functions related to education and training.
         b. Food and Drug Administration helps ensure the safety and efficacy of food, pharmaceuticals, and other consumer goods.
         c. Health Resources and Service Administration develops health programs, services, and facilities for certain populations such as Native Americans and federal prisoners.
         d. National Institutes of Health (NIH) supports research programs, largely by providing funding.
         e. Alcohol, Drug Abuse, and Mental Health Administration supports research and programs related to substance abuse and mental health.
         f. Agency for Toxic Substances and Disease Registry works to prevent adverse health effects from hazardous substances in the environment.
   B. Scope and focus
      1. The federal government focuses on the health of the general population and on special populations such as veterans, Native Americans, and federal prisoners. It also focuses on the international community.
      2. The federal government directs efforts to improve health habits and to prevent the use of tobacco, drugs, and alcohol. It also offers programs to improve nutrition.

V. **Roles of the State Government in Public Health**
   A. Organization
      1. States are responsible for the health of their citizens, but organization varies greatly from state to state.
         a. Some states have a health officer who is in charge of all programs.
         b. Other states have boards of health.
      2. Nurses are the largest group of professionals providing services at the state level.
   B. Scope and focus
      1. The scope of public health varies greatly from state to state.
      2. Most states include three basic types of services.
         a. Assessment—epidemiological activities, laboratory analyses, participation in research projects, and data collection for vital statistics
         b. Policy development—formulation of goals, development of health plans, and setting of standards for local agencies
         c. Assurance activities—inspection, licensing, health education, environmental safety, and resource development

VI. **Roles of the Local Government in Public Health**
   A. Organization of local health departments
      1. Health department is responsible for direct delivery of public health services to citizens.
      2. Local services vary greatly from community to community, depending largely on resources, geographic size, and population.
   B. Scope
      1. Responsibilities of local health departments
         a. Determine the health status and needs of its constituents
         b. Identify unmet needs
         c. Take action to meet needs
      2. Most services for groups and individuals at the local level fall into four categories.
         a. Environmental health services—inspection of food production and restaurants, protection for hazardous substances, control of waste, and pollution control)
         b. Community health services—control of communicable disease through surveillance and immunization, maternal/child programs, and education
         c. Mental health services—focus on primary prevention, diagnosis, and treatment
         d. Personal health care—care to individuals in clinics, schools, jails, and homes

VII. Future of the Health Care System
  A. Changes and influences in the health care system will be necessary for many reasons
    1. Increasing incidence of chronic illnesses such as AIDS and cancer
    2. Environmental hazards
    3. Aging of the population
    4. Increased consumer involvement
    5. Escalating health care costs
    6. Increased technology
    7. Fewer hospital admissions
  B. Health care financing
    1. The current system is pluralistic and competitive.
    2. The current system provides fragmented, uncoordinated care. Services by one agency or provider do not help the patient move across organizations or receive the services of others.
    3. The focus of service has not kept pace with the changing needs of individuals and populations.
    4. Currently, 40 million Americans do not have health insurance, and an additional 33 million are served by Medicaid.
    5. The majority of health care dollars go toward diagnosis and treatment rather than prevention.
    6. During the 1980s, the social policy changed from improving access to containing costs.
  C. Cost containment
    1. In the past, services were provided based on the medical model and focused more on treatment than on prevention.
    2. Diagnostic practice and treatment usually depended on the most sophisticated technology. Laboratory tests and diagnostic tests and treatments increased the cost of care dramatically.
    3. In the mid-late 1990s, there has been a sense of urgency for health care organizations and providers to join networks of care.
    4. Cost containment through managed care has become the fastest growing movement in the 1990s. "Managed care" can refer to an HMO (Kaiser-Permanente) or an affiliation of physicians and hospitals linked by another organization (usually an insurance company).

  D. State initiatives in health care reform
    1. State reform initiatives usually focus on services to publicly sponsored residents.
    2. Movement of these patients to managed care arrangements has begun. In these settings, greater emphasis is placed on health promotion and cost containment.
  E. The Clinton health reform initiative
    1. Support for health care reform was high in the early 1990s.
    2. Initially, the process was supported by many service providers (businesses, physicians, hospitals), but many withdrew support as the process progressed.
    3. The insurance industry sector was the most opposed to reform.
  F. A return to reform at the state level
    1. Due to the failure of the Clinton health care initiative, reform efforts were enhanced at the state level.
    2. The concept of combining categorical funds into block grants is becoming common.
    3. Reducing the role of the national government by sending federal health and medical programs to the states as block grants has affected the funding of community-based public health programs.
  G. Future of public health and the health care system—It is clear that the community health focus on health promotion and disease prevention and the population-based approach to health care provision will increase in the future.

TEACHING STRATEGIES

  1. If the local public health department is not a routinely used clinical site, arrange for a visit by the class. Encourage the public health officials (ideally nurses) to explain the services provided by the health department.
  2. Invite guest speakers from various DHHS agencies to discuss services provided by their agency. For example, officers from the U.S. Public Health Service can describe the wide variety of services they offer; officials from the Health Care Financing Administration can discuss the impact of DRGs on health care, or individuals from the Office of Human Development Services can describe program planning.

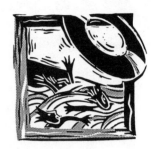

CHAPTER 4

Thinking Upstream: Conceptualizing Health from a Population Perspective

ANNOTATED LEARNING OBJECTIVES

1. **Describe the concept of theoretic scope as it applies to the protection and promotion of health in community health nursing.**

   The term *theoretic scope* refers to the range or perspective taken by the nurse in assessing and analyzing a health problem and planning appropriate interventions. Theory is used to improve nursing practice by guiding data collection and interpretation. Theoretic scope determines whether these efforts are microscopic or macroscopic.

   Traditional, individual-based nursing care is microscopic in nature. It focuses on the individual and one or two immediate health concerns.

   The macroscopic approach is comprehensive. Nursing tasks such as data collection, data analysis, and planning take environmental, demographic, social, and economic factors into consideration. The macroscopic approach, when applied to community health nursing, allows the nurse to consider these factors when determining the health needs of the population and planning health promotion and protection interventions.

2. **Differentiate between upstream interventions, which are designed to alter the precursors of poor health, and downstream interventions, which are characterized by efforts to modify individuals' perceptions of their health.**

   Upstream and downstream interventions can be differentiated using an analogy of victims in a river. Downstream interventions focus on correcting the problem after it has occurred. The victim has already fallen in the river; downstream interventions "pull the victim out."

   Downstream interventions are characterized by short-term, individual-based interventions.

Examples include testing, treating, and providing education about tuberculosis.

   Upstream interventions, on the other hand, focus on preventing the problem before it happens. In other words, upstream interventions try to find out "what is pushing the victims into the river" and then take measures to prevent it.

   Upstream interventions focus on modification of economic, political, and environmental factors to improve the health of the community. Examples of upstream interventions include identification of aggregates at risk for development of tuberculosis; instituting measures to improve living conditions and nutrition for those at risk; and encouraging continuing research for new drugs to prevent and treat tuberculosis. These efforts are designed to alter factors that determine poor health prior to disease.

3. **Critique a theory in regard to its relevance to facilitating an understanding of population health dynamics.**

   This chapter presents four theories and describes their application to population-based nursing. Orem's Self-Care Deficit Theory and the Health Belief Model are narrow in scope and therefore are more appropriate to directing individual intervention, as opposed to community or aggregate intervention.

   Critical Social Theory and Milio's Framework for Prevention are much broader in scope and can help the community health nurse understand and facilitate community-based health promotion and protection interventions.

4. **Recognize theory-based practice as the means of meeting community health nursing's responsibilities to protect and promote health in populations.**

   The goal of theory is to improve nursing by guiding nursing practice. Theory-based practice guides the process of data collection and interpretation and facilitates appropriate problem diagnoses and the planning of interventions for identified problems. In community health nursing, the application of appropriate theories and theoretical concepts enables the nurse to diagnose accurately threats and potential threats to population health. Theory-based practice helps the nurse determine proven, effective, appropriate interventions designed to promote health and prevent illness in those populations.

LECTURE OUTLINE

I. **Thinking Upstream: Looking Beyond the Individual**—This analogy describes how health care workers are caught up with "rescuing victims from the river."
- A. *Downstream* endeavors
  1. Analogous to "pulling the victims out of the river"
  2. Characterized by short-term, individual-based interventions
- B. *Upstream* endeavors
  1. Analogous to "looking upstream to identify what is pushing the victims into the river"
  2. Characterized by a focus on modifying economic, political, and environmental factors to improve health.

II. **Historic Perspectives on Nursing Theory**
- A. Florence Nightingale was the first nurse to formulate a conceptual foundation for nursing practice.
- B. After Florence Nightingale, nursing practice was defined primarily by hospital administrative and medical personnel.
- C. In an effort to regain control of nursing theory and practice, nursing leaders began to advance nursing through development of theories.

III. **Issues of Fit**
- A. Nurses must learn to use theory appropriately. They must learn not to "force fit" a situation into a theory or a theory onto a situation.
- B. To utilize theory to guide community health nursing practice, the nurse should select theoretic approaches that are compatible with a population perspective.

IV. **Definitions of Theory**
- A. Nursing definitions of theory lack uniformity. They reflect differences in conceptualization among research, theory, and practice.
- B. Common themes among definitions of theory
  1. A set of concepts, propositions, or relational statements
  2. A framework or system
  3. An end or purpose

V. **Theory to What End?**
- A. The goal of using theory is to guide, and thereby improve, the practice of nursing.
- B. Theory-based practice guides data collection and interpretation in a clear and organized manner.

VI. **Microscopic vs. Macroscopic Approaches to the Conceptualization of Community Health Problems**
- A. Typically, nurses and other health care providers take a *microscopic* perspective that focuses exclusively on the individual and one or two problems.
  1. Interventions are planned on an individual basis.
  2. In an archery analogy, the microscopic approach targets only the "bull's-eye."
- B. A *macroscopic* approach is comprehensive.
  1. The nurse considers environmental, demographic, social, and economic factors when planning intervention.
  2. The macroscopic approach targets both the bull's-eye and the surrounding concentric circles for intervention.

VII. **Scope of Theory in Community Health Nursing**
- A. Most nursing theories focus on the individual.
- B. Unless a given theory is macroscopic and addresses health and determinants of health from a population perspective, it is of limited use to community health nurses.

VIII. **Microscopic Theories**
- A. *Orem's Self-Care Deficit Theory of Nursing* is based on the premise that nursing is a response to one's incapacity to care for one's self because of one's health.
  1. Nursing assumes the role of providing some or all self-care activities on behalf of the patient.
  2. The concepts of self-care, self-care deficit, and self-care agency are microscopic in nature and difficult to apply to populations.
- B. The *Health Belief Model* resulted from the desire to understand factors that influence preventive health behaviors.
  1. An assumption of the model is that the major determinant of preventive health behavior is the avoidance of disease.
  2. The model was not designed to be generalized across disorders, so actions that relate to preventive health behaviors for each disease differ from one another.

3. The Health Belief Model is narrow in scope.
    a. It places the burden of action exclusively on the client.
    b. It assumes that only clients who have negative perceptions of the specified disease or recommended health action will fail to act.
4. Interventions are generally focused on the alteration of a patient's perspectives and are based on the individual.

IX. **Macroscopic Theories**
  A. *Milio's Framework for Prevention* provides for the inclusion of economic, political, and environmental health determinants and is broad in range.
    1. Milio's framework relates the ability of an individual to improve healthful behavior to society's ability to provide options for healthy choices that are accessible and socially desirable.
    2. The range of choices available is shaped by government and private policy decision.
    3. Health deficits result from an imbalance between a population's health needs and its health-sustaining resources.
    4. To improve health status, health-promoting choices must be readily available and less costly than health-damaging options.
    5. The range of health-promoting or health-damaging choices available to individuals is affected by their personal resources (awareness, knowledge and beliefs, money, time, and other priorities) and societal resources (availability and cost of health services, environmental protection, shelter).
  B. *Critical Social Theory* is based on the belief that life is structured by social meanings that are determined through social domination.
    1. Critical Social Theory assumes that standards of truth are determined socially.
    2. Application of Critical Social Theory necessitates inductive reasoning in which the nurse assesses concepts through an ongoing process of data collection and analysis.
    3. Politico-economic interventions are the most effective method of addressing the health of a population; these interventions seek to eliminate illness at the source.
    4. Critical Social Theory holds each person responsible for creating social conditions in which all members of society are able to speak freely. Nurses are thereby challenged to expose power imbalances that prohibit people from achieving their full potential.

TEACHING STRATEGIES

1. Make a transparency of the "Definitions of Theory" table using the box supplied in the text. Have students compare and contrast the various definitions and relate how they apply to community health nursing.
2. Assign students to present briefly and then discuss one or two nursing theories. Ask students to critique the relevance of each theory to population-focused (macroscopic) interventions.

Community Assessment and Epidemiology

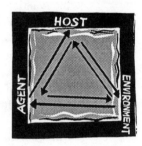

ANNOTATED LEARNING OBJECTIVES

1. *Discuss the major dimensions of a community.*

   Communities are composed of people, geographic or physical locations, and social systems. The people within a community share one or more common characteristics, such as interests, concerns, goals, activities, or heredity. Communities may be defined on the basis of geographic or physical location. Geopolitical definitions include cities, counties, and school districts. Examples of communities with non-geopolitical definitions include dormitories, tenement buildings, and worksites, among others. A community is a social system with interacting members comprising interrelated and interdependent subsystems within the community.

2. *Identify the major sources of information about a community's health.*

   Sources of data for assessing a community's health include:

   Census—provides information about each household, including age, sex, race, socioeconomic status, housing characteristics, and education.

   Vital Statistics—official records of births, deaths, marriages, divorces, and adoptions; can be obtained from city, county, state, and federal sources.

   National Center for Health Statistics—compiles information about disability, illnesses, and other health-related variables.

   Local and state health departments and agencies—provide information about the health of the community.

3. *Use epidemiological methods to describe the state of health of a community or aggregate.*

   Following the collection of health-related data, rates are calculated to describe the health of the community. Rates are expressed as proportions or fractions and are used to interpret raw data and to make comparisons among aggregates or communities. Incidence rates describe the occurrence of new disease cases in a community over a period of time. Prevalence rates describe the number of all cases of a disease in a population at a point in time. Crude rates and variable-specific rates are also used to describe populations.

4. *Identify epidemiological study designs for researching health problems.*

   A number of epidemiological study designs are useful in examining health problems. These include:

   Cross-sectional (prevalence or correlational) studies—establish correlations between variables and disease; generate hypotheses for further study.

   Retrospective (case control) studies—compare groups of individuals that have a disease with similar groups that do not have the disease. Data collection extends back in time to determine previous exposure or risk factors.

   Prospective (longitudinal or cohort) studies—follow groups of individuals who are disease-free for an extended period of time. Exposure to factors suspective of disease association is assessed, and groups exposed to these factors are compared to those who are not.

   Experimental studies—require the investigator to assign subjects to experimental and control groups, manipulate one or more variables, and observe the occurrence of disease in each group. Experimental studies are useful for determining causality.

5. *Formulate aggregate diagnoses.*

   An aggregate diagnosis has four components: an identified health risk, an aggregate or community that is affected, an etiological or causal statement, and evidence or support for the diagnosis. Examples are:

- Increased risk of sexually transmitted disease among students at Johnson High School related to limited understanding of STD transmission and prevention and high rates of sexual activity as demonstrated by an increase in the number of Johnson students reporting to the school nurse and county clinic.

- Increased risk of tuberculosis among homeless individuals in New York City related to poor nutrition, living conditions conducive to transmission, and increased potential for exposure as demonstrated by reported increases in incidence rate for TB in New York City, the state of New York, and the United States.

LECTURE OUTLINE

Community- or population-focused practice requires the ability to apply the nursing process to meet the health needs of groups, aggregates, and populations. To provide health services, the community health nurse often must consider the community itself as the unit of service.

I.   **The Nature of a Community**
  A. A community is composed of people who share one or more common characteristics.
    1. In a community, people share interests and concerns, and they often have common goals and activities.
    2. People in a community may share health traits or *risk factors* that predispose them to disease or impaired health.
    3. When individuals come together because of a common problem, a *community of solution* is formed.
  B. Communities may be defined on the basis of geographic or physical location.
    1. Geopolitical boundaries include city limits, census tracts, voting precincts, school districts, etc.
    2. Non-geopolitical boundaries include neighborhoods, dormitories, tenement buildings, summer camps, etc.
  C. A community is a social system with interacting members comprising subsystems within the community. The subsystems are interrelated and interdependent.
  D. Residents can claim membership in several communities simultaneously.

II. **Assessing the Community: Sources of Data**
  A. *Census data* are gathered every ten years by the U.S. Bureau of the Census.

    1. The census provides demographic information, including age, gender, race, ethnicity, education, socioeconomic status, and housing characteristics of each member of a census tract.
    2. A census tract is a small area of 3000 to 6000 people, most of whom share similar characteristics (ethnicity, socioeconomic status, and housing type).
    3. Variables that describe the health of the community are not part of the census data. Census information allows comparison of data from one community with that of other communities and with data from previous time periods. These comparisons are essential in analysis and interpretation of the data.
  B. *Vital statistics* are the official registration records of births, deaths, marriages, divorces, and adoptions.
    1. These events are collected and reported annually by city, county, and state health departments.
    2. Like the census data, vital statistics are compared for analysis and diagnosis of problems and potential problems.
  C. The *National Center for Health Statistics* distributes prevalence reports of disability, illness, and other health-related variables.
  D. *Local and state agencies* can be valuable sources of health data about a community.

III. **Assessing the Community: The Use of Rates**
  A. Rates are used to facilitate and interpret raw data and to make comparisons.
    1. Rates are written as proportions or fractions in which the numerator is the number of events that occur in a specified period of time.
    2. By converting raw counts to rates, the community health nurse can make meaningful comparisons with rates from other districts, states, or the entire nation.
    3. Rates also make possible meaningful comparisons with a previous time period.
    4. For more information, see Appendix A: "Calculation of Morbidity and Mortality Rates."
  B. One of the two principal types of morbidity rates (rates of illness) is the incidence rate.
    1. *Incidence rates* describe the occurrence of new disease cases in a community over a period of time relative to the size of the population at risk of developing that disease during that period.

2. Incidence rates are particularly useful for detecting short-term, acute disease changes.
3. The *attack rate* is a special incidence rate that documents the number of new cases of a disease in those exposed to a disease.

C. The other principal type of morbidity rate is the prevalence rate.
   1. The *prevalence rate* is the number of all cases of a specific disease in a population at a given point in time relative to the population at risk of acquiring the disease at the same point in time.
   2. Prevalence rates are influenced by the number of people who develop the particular condition (incidence) and the duration of the condition. An increase in the incidence rate or the duration of a disease increases the prevalence rate of that disease.

D. Other rates are also useful in characterizing populations.
   1. *Crude rates* summarize the occurrence of births (crude birth rate) or deaths (crude death rate). The numerator is the number of events, and the denominator is the average population size. Crude rates may contain biases because the denominator is the total population rather than the population at risk.
   2. *Age-specific rates* are used to overcome some of the biases seen with crude rates. Similar rates may also be used to control for other variables such as race and gender.
   3. *Age-adjustment* or *standardized rates* reduce bias due to unequivalent age distribution of the populations being compared.
   4. The *proprtionate mortality rate (PMR)* represents the percentage of deaths resulting from a specific cause relative to deaths from all causes.

IV. **Epidemiology**
A. Epidemiology is the study of the distribution and determinants of health and disease in the community. It is the principal science of community health practice.
B. Epidemiology permits identification of factors critical to the development of disease. Examination of characteristics of disease in terms of person, place, and time allows epidemiologists to identify relationships between determinants of disease.
C. Three common models of epidemiology
   1. The epidemiological triangle
      a. This model is used to analyze disease development dependent on exposure to an agent, the host's susceptibility, and the environmental conditions existing at the time of exposure.
      b. The triangle is applicable to conditions that can be linked to clearly identifiable agents.
   2. The wheel model
      a. This model consists of a hub and a surrounding wheel. The hub represents the host with its human characteristics (genetics, immunity, and personality).
      b. The wheel surrounding the hub represents the environment and is composed of biological, social, and physical dimensions.
      c. The relative size of each component in the wheel depends on the health problem being analyzed.
      d. Because the wheel allows for a multiple-causation theory of disease, it is useful for analyzing complex chronic conditions.
   3. The web of causation
      a. This model illustrates the complexity of the interaction of risk factors that can lead to the development of chronic illness.
      b. The web of causation is useful in the development of interventions to address identified risk factors.

D. Use of epidemiology in secondary and tertiary prevention
   1. *Establishing causality*—Disease causality cannot be proven definitively; however, it may be established in terms of a strong association or identified causal factors. The following criteria are needed to determine a cause-and-effect relationship.
      a. *Strength of association*—Rates of morbidity and mortality must be higher in the exposed group than in the non-exposed group.
      b. *Dose-response relationship*—As exposure to a risk factor increases, there must be a concomitant increase in the disease rate.
      c. *Temporally correct relationship*—Exposure to the risk factor must occur before the effect (disease).
      d. *Biological plausibility*—The data must provide a coherent explanation for the relationship.
      e. *Consistency with other studies*—Similar associations must have been made in other studies and other populations.

f. *Specificity*—The exposure to the risk factor must be necessary and sufficient to cause the disease.
2. *Screening*—The purpose of screening programs is to identify risk factors and diseases in their earliest stages. Screening is usually classified as a secondary prevention activity because disease is discovered after a pathologic change has occurred. Guidelines for screening programs include:
   a. Adequate and appropriate followup should be planned for those who test positive.
   b. Early diagnosis of the disease should be beneficial.
   c. Acceptable and medically sound treatment should be available.
   d. Procedures for ensuring confidentiality should be in place.
   e. Tests must be cost-effective and acceptable to the client.
   f. Costs of the program, followup, and resulting medical care should have a bearing on the decision to screen.
   g. Screening tests should ideally have a high *sensitivity* (the ability to detect people who have the disease) and *specificity* (the ability to identify people who do not have the disease).
3. *Surveillance*—Surveillance allows ongoing collection of information by monitoring changes in disease frequency and trends in occurrence of risk factors. The nurse evaluates trends in morbidity by identifying new cases and calculating incidence rates.
E. Use of epidemiology in health services
   1. Epidemiology is useful in studying the delivery of health care to populations by describing and evaluating the use of health services by the community.
   2. Epidemiological studies can be used to evaluate quality of care.

V. **Types of Epidemiology**
   A. Descriptive epidemiology
      1. Focuses on the distribution of health problems within a population and on the effects of person, place, and time factors on an illness
      2. Describes the characteristics of people who are protected from specific diseases and of those who have specific diseases
      3. Variables in descriptive epidemiology include age, gender, ethnicity or race, socioeconomic status, occupation, education, and family status

   B. Analytic epidemiology
      1. Investigates the causes of disease by determining why a disease rate is lower in one population group than in another.
      2. Generates and tests hypotheses from descriptive data to establish a cause-and-effect relationship between a preexisting condition or event and the disease
      3. Uses observational and/or experimental research studies to determine causal relationships

VI. **Epidemiological Methods**
   A. Cross-sectional (prevalence or correlational) studies
      1. Examine relationships between potential causal factors and disease at a point in time
      2. Are primarily hypothesis-generating tools used to identify preliminary relationships for further exploration
      3. Are of limited value in establishing etiological factors of disease
   B. Retrospective (case control) studies
      1. Retrospective studies compare a group of individuals known to have a disease with a similar group of individuals who do not have the disease.
      2. The purpose is to determine whether the diseased group differs from the nondiseased control group in its exposure to a specific factor or characteristic.
      3. Data collection extends back in time to determine previous exposure or risk factors.
      4. Retrospective studies can address the question of causality and require fewer resources and less time for data collection than other types of studies.
   C. Prospective (longitudinal or cohort) studies
      1. These studies identify a group of individuals considered to be free of disease and follow them forward in time to determine if and when disease occurs.
      2. The cohort (group of people who share a common experience within a defined time period) is assessed for exposure factors suspected of being associated with a disease. The cohort is then followed for the development of disease.
      3. The disease rates for those with a known exposure are compared with the rates for those who remain unexposed, and incidence and relative risk are determined.
      4. Prospective studies provide reliable information about the etiology of disease, but they are very costly and time-consuming.

D. Experimental studies
1. Experimental studies require the investigator to assign subjects who are at risk randomly to an experimental or control group. Only the experimental group is subject to the intervention, but both groups are observed over time for occurrence of the disease.
2. Ethical considerations prohibit the use of human subjects in many experiments. Experimental studies are therefore generally restricted to clinical trials of prophylactic and therapeutic measures.

VII. **Application of the Nursing Process**
A. The synthesis of assessment data into diagnostic statements about the health of the community is the second step of the nursing process. These statements specify the nature and etiology of the actual or potential community health problem. They also direct plans developed by the community health nurse to resolve the problem.
B. A community nursing diagnosis consists of four components.
1. Health problem or risk
2. Aggregate or community affected
3. Etiological or causal statement
4. Evidence or support for the diagnosis

TEACHING STRATEGIES

1. Divide the class into groups of four or five students. Using the "Community Assessment Parameters Guide" in the text, have students do a community assessment on a community or aggregate of their choice. They may choose a census tract, rural community, dormitory, or other aggregate. If students are able to collect data on vital statistics, have them calculate rates such as birth and death rates, cause-specific death rates, and rate of teenage pregnancy.
2. Using the community diagnosis outline provided, create a transparency. Have students discuss problems they have identified in the community and practice writing aggregate or community diagnoses.
3. Using the data and the formulas provided, have students calculate birth and death rates for several census tracts. Compare the rates of the tracts with each other and with that of the state.
4. Have students search health care journals for examples of epidemiological research studies. In groups, have them classify each study as descriptive, cross-sectional, retrospective, prospective, or experimental. Attempt to find examples of each type of study.

Community Health Planning and Evaluation

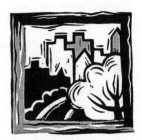

ANNOTATED LEARNING OBJECTIVES

1. Define what is meant by "aggregate as client."

"Aggregate as client" refers to the focus of health care planning and intervention on groups, aggregates, organizations, or communities instead of on individuals and families.

2. Apply the nursing process within a systems framework to the larger aggregate.

Using the health planning model (described below), the nurse can assess, plan, intervene, and evaluate an actual or potential health need of a group or aggregate. Systems are characterized by structure, functions, and process. The nurse must realize that systems continually interact with, and adapt to, the environment. Within a system, assessment is ongoing. Interventions should be goal-directed, and evaluation data must be incorporated into continual planning.

3. Describe the steps in the health planning model.

Assessment—In the assessment phase, the nurse (1) gathers information regarding sociodemographic characteristics of the aggregate; (2) performs a literature review to compare the aggregate with the "norm"; and (3) identifies and prioritizes health needs or problems. It is important to consider the needs perceived by the aggregate when identifying and prioritizing health needs.

Planning—Planning should be based on the prioritization of real or potential health problems. The nurse (1) determines specific and measurable goals; (2) identifies the appropriate levels of intervention (individual, aggregate, community); (3) considers the practicality of the interventions, given available personnel and aggregate resources; and (4) schedules the plan with the aggregate.

Intervention—During the intervention step, the nurse implements at least one level of the plan. The nurse should prepare to be flexible and to alter the plans if necessary.

Evaluation—Evaluation of a program should be based on the objectives of the program, the plan for implementing it, and the actual outcomes observed. To evaluate, the nurse collects data from participants and determines the strengths and weaknesses of the plan, considering both positive and negative aspects of the program.

4. Identify the level of prevention and the system level appropriate for nursing interventions with aggregates.

After identifying the source of the problem, the nurse should determine the appropriate system level(s), (subsystem, aggregate system, and/or suprasystem) for direction of intervention. Is the source of the health problem one that can best be addressed at the individual, family, group, aggregate, or community level?

5. Compare and contrast goals and outcomes of health planning legislation from the Hill-Burton Act to the National Health Planning and Resources Development Act.

Compare—The Hill-Burton Act (1946), the Heart Disease, Cancer, and Stroke Amendments of 1965, the Public Health Service Act Amendments (1966), and the National Health Planning and Resources Development Act (1974) were all needs-based efforts to improve access to quality health care, thereby improving health.

Contrast—Hill-Burton funded hospital construction and modernization based on state-wide planning; it was very helpful in providing care to rural areas. The Heart Disease, Cancer, and Stroke Amendment was a regional effort that developed medical centers to provide the "latest technology"; it led to duplication of services in many areas. The Public Health Service Act mandated consumer involvement and was opposed by many providers. The National Health Planning and Resources Development Act focused on single-state health planning agencies to increase accessibility and acceptability, reduce costs, and prevent duplication of health resources.

6. Identify the advantages of comprehensive health planning and evaluation.

Comprehensive health planning is designed to promote and ensure high levels of health for everyone. Potential advantages of comprehensive health planning and evaluation include encouragement of consumer involvement, accessibility, acceptability, continuity and quality of health service, prevention of duplication of health resources, and cost reduction.

7. Describe the community health nurse's role in health planning and evaluation.

Increased nursing involvement will strengthen local and national health planning. The community health nurse identifies health needs and subsequently plans, implements, and evaluates interventions. Emphasizing the aggregate as client improves the health of individuals and families.

LECTURE OUTLINE

I. **Overview of Health Planning**
   A. Early public health nursing efforts incorporated nurses' visits to people in their homes with application of the nursing process to larger aggregates and communities to improve the health of a greater number of people.
   B. In the mid-1960s, the focus shifted from the aggregate to the individual and family, where it remains today.
   C. During the mid-1980s, community health nurses recognized the need to reemphasize aggregate and community care. Information about communities can help nurses understand the health problems of individuals and families. To accomplish health promotion and disease prevention efforts for entire communities, health planning at the aggregate or community level is necessary.

II. **Health Planning Model**—The health planning model applies the nursing process to an aggregate within a systems framework to improve the health of the aggregate. It can help the nurse gain knowledge and experience in the the health planning process.

A. *Assessment*—During the assessment phase of the nursing process the nurse gathers information from several sources. To do this, the nurse must first establish a professional relationship and meet with members of the aggregate or with individuals or groups who will work with the aggregate. Good communication skills are essential. The following activities are included in the assessment phase of the nursing process.
   1. The nurse collects information regarding sociodemographic characteristics.
      a. These may be gathered from a variety of sources, including observation, consultation, record review, or interview of aggregate members.
      b. The nurse must consider both positive and negative factors.
      c. The nurse assesses the suprasystem in which the aggregate is located, including support services and facilities.
      d. Assessment may require exploring public records and talking with health professionals, volunteers, and key informants.
   2. The nurse performs a literature review to compare the aggregate with the "norm."
   3. The nurse identifies and prioritizes the health problems and/or needs of the specific aggregate.
      a. The nurse analyzes the assessment data and compares it with the information from the literature review.
      b. It is very important at this step for the nurse to incorporate the aggregate members' perception of the need(s).
      c. To prioritize health problems and needs, the nurse must consider several factors.
         1) The aggregate's preference
         2) The number of individuals affected by the problem
         3) The severity of the health need
         4) The availability of potential solutions
         5) Practical considerations such as skills, time limitations, and available resources
      d. Assessment is ongoing throughout the process. Planning should stem directly from it and should be realistic in terms of implementation.
B. *Planning*—Planning should be based on prioritization of real or potential health problems. The ultimate goal should be identified at this stage of the process. Goals and objectives must be specific and measurable. The planning phase includes the following steps.

1. Determine the level or levels (subsystem, aggregate system, and/or suprasystem) at which inteventions will be planned.
2. Plan interventions for each system level that will accomplish the objectives. Interventions may be at any of the three levels of prevention—primary, secondary, or tertiary.
3. Validate the practicality of the interventions, given the available personal, aggregate, and suprasystem resources.
4. Plan the scheduling of the interventions with the aggregate.
C. *Intervention*—Plans for interventions should proceed as set forth, but the nurse should be prepared to be flexible enough to deal with unexpected contingencies.
D. *Evaluation*—In the evaluation phase, the nurse considers the outcomes of the interventions. Were the stated goals met? Evaluation includes three activities.
   1. Collect data, or feedback, from participants
   2. Reflect on each previous stage to determine strengths and weaknesses of the process
   3. Address both positive and negative aspects of the project

III. **Health Planning Projects**
A. Health planning projects should be designed to intervene with different types of aggregates, groups, organizations, or communities at one of the three systems levels (subsystem, aggregate system, or suprasystem).
B. Projects should address a particular level of prevention. Most interventions are primary prevention and occur at the individual level.
C. Successful projects apply the nursing process to aggregates, groups, and populations by employing a variety of interventions.
D. Lack of success of a project is often related to problems identified at one or more steps of the nursing process.
   1. Incomplete assessment
   2. Failure to identify key informants
   3. Failure to identify mutual goals and objectives
   4. Uncontrollable or unanticipated events or circumstances
E. Summary of health planning projects
   1. Health planning projects should target all three levels of prevention at a variety of systems levels.
   2. Assessment should be thorough and include a comparison of the aggregate's health and demographic information with that of similar aggregates in the literature.

3. Planning should include mutual identification and setting of goals and objectives.
4. Implementation of interventions must include aggregate participation and must be goal-oriented.
5. In the evaluation phase, both the process and the outcome of the intervention must be evaluated. Input from the aggregate is essential.

IV. **Health Planning Legislation**
A. Early efforts at health planning were usually initiated by private, nongovernment agencies. The federal government became involved at the end of World War II. The government acted because of a general shortage of hospital beds, particularly in rural areas.
B. Congress passed the Hill-Burton Act (Hospital Survey and Construction Act) in 1946 to provide federal aid to states for hospital construction and modernization. Eligibility for funds was based on a plan submitted by the state. The number of available hospital beds increased, mostly in general hospitals.
C. The Heart Disease, Cancer, and Stroke Amendments (1965) established regional medical programs to make technology available to community health care providers. Fifty-six health regions were established to evaluate the health needs within each regon.
D. The Public Health Service Act Amendments (1966) created the "Partnership for Health Program."
   1. This program was meant to promote and ensure the highest level of health attainable for every person.
   2. The plans were designed to encourage consumer involvement, but they were opposed by many providers (the American Medical Association, American Hospital Association, and major medical centers), and therefore were not successful in accomplishing their goals.
E. In the mid-1960s, many states began to require a *certificate of need* to control health care costs and expenditures more effectively. The "need" for the planned project or expenditure must be determined and approved by the state prior to certain major capital expenditures by hospitals and nursing homes.
F. The National Health Planning and Resources Development Act (1974) was written to encourage development of single-state health planning agencies. Only marginal success has been achieved.

1. Its primary goal was to increase accessibility, acceptability, continuity, and quality of health services. Other goals were to prevent duplication of health resources and reduce the costs of health services.
2. It created a network of local health planning agencies. Each agency developed a health systems plan for a geographic service area.

G. During the 1980s, competition within the health care system was encouraged.
   1. Emphasis was placed on cost shifting and cost containment.
   2. Federal health planning programs suffered cutbacks in funding.

H. During the 1990s, comprehensive plans have been undertaken at the state and local levels to provide improved care at lower costs. Implementation of "managed care" programs and strategies are increasingly directing health planning and cost management.

V. **Nursing Implications**

A. Increased nursing involvement will serve to strengthen local, state, and national health planning.

B. Identification of health needs of the aggregate, with subsequent planning, intervention, and evaluation, will improve the health of individuals and families.

TEACHING STRATEGIES

1. Obtain copies of several comprehensive health plans such as *Healthy People 2000* and the 1990 *Health Objectives for the Nation,* as well as plans from local and state health departments. Discuss components of each plan with students. Do they include assessment data, analysis, written goals and objectives, plans, etc.? Have the plans been implemented? Is any evaluation data available?

2. Have students plan a health program using the "Health Planning Project Objectives—Guide" in the textbook. The aggregate can be actual (identified from clinical experiences) or hypothetical (anticipated from the literature or personal experiences).

3. Invite an administrator from the local, regional, or state health department to speak to the class regarding program planning at the community or state level.

Community Organization: Building Partnerships for Health

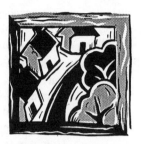

ANNOTATED LEARNING OBJECTIVES

1. Define community organization, community development, social planning, and social action.

Community organization is the process by which community change agents such as nurses empower individuals and aggregates to solve community problems and achieve community goals.

Community development is a community organization model that emphasizes community involvement, self-direction, and self-help in determining and solving problems.

Social planning is a model in which community decisions are based on fact gathering and rational decision making. Emphasis is placed on the task rather than the process. It is the model most universally supported by nursing theories.

Social action is the model in which community change is accomplished by polarization of the community around an issue, followed by confrontation or conflict between people who have opposing viewpoints.

2. Explain major concepts, models, theoretical frameworks, and strategies of community organization.

Concepts of community organization include systems theories, social change, and community participation. Models of community organization include social planning, social action, and community development models. Strategies for community organization include collaboration, campaign, and contest strategies.

3. Discuss the relationships among community health development, social justice, and nursing care of aggregates.

Access to basic health care for all people is a social justice concern and a community health

nursing goal. Community health development refers to the process by which community organizations work to identify health-related needs, set goals, and work to meet those goals.

4. Describe strategies for building community partnerships for health promotion and disease and injury prevention.

Strategies for building community organizations for health promotion include campaign strategies, contest strategies, and collaboration strategies.

Using a social planning model, the nurse might need to apply campaign strategies. These strategies are useful when people within an aggregate have different opinions about an issue or solution, but the possibility of consensus still exists. In social planning, the nurse collects data to identify major problems and groups at risk. Decisions are based on assessment data. Roles of the nurse include facilitator, fact gatherer, analyst, and program implementor.

Using a social action model, the nurse may use contest strategies to address inequities in health and health care. Contest strategies are appropriate when existing power structures in a community fail to recognize a problem or strongly oppose a proposed solution. Social action stresses that confrontation and conflict can be employed to achieve desired health goals. Nursing roles in the social action model include community activist, agitator, and negotiator.

Collaboration strategies are used by community health nurses with a community development model when there is consensus and basic agreement on an issue or problem. Active participation, self-direction, and self-help by the aggregate are encouraged. The nurse acts as an enabler and teacher or educator of problem-solving skills.

LECTURE OUTLINE

According to the ANA, a major responsibility of community health nurses is to act as advocate for individuals and families by identifying and rectifying gaps in health care services and influencing health and social policies that are inconsistent with health care. One way to achieve this is through removal of barriers such as distance, lack of transportation, time, lack of knowledge, lack of coordinated care, and lack of services appropriate to culture, religion, or language.

I. **Conceptual Basis of Community Organization**
   A. Social systems theories
      1. Communities are systems that have wholeness, boundaries, organization, openness, and feedback.
      2. Communities consist of interrelated subsystems composed of aggregates (groups that share common characteristics) and sectors (functional divisions of the community, such as health, welfare, education, economics, energy, religion, communication, business, and recreation).
      3. In systems theory, all sectors and aggregates are interrelated. A change in one subsystem affects all other subsystems as well as the community as a whole.
      4. Specific theories
         a. Neuman's health-care systems model is a social systems theory.
         b. Anderson and McFarlane's community-as-client model presents an integrated system-oriented framework for community health nursing practice.
   B. Social change
      1. The process of social change has three stages.
         a. Unfreezing
         b. Changing
         c. Refreezing
      2. Change is affected by driving and restraining forces that promote or oppose a proposed change.
      3. Change occurs when the strength or direction of the driving forces and/or restraining forces is changed.
   C. Community participation
      1. Community participation is a variable associated with health communities.
         a. *Participatory change* occurs when members of the aggregate are involved in planning and problem solving at all levels of change.
         b. *Directive change* is imposed on the community by outside forces.
      2. A *coalition* is a group of diverse agencies, organizations, and individuals that work together to address a common interest or concern. Coalition formation is a useful strategy for community participation.
      3. *Community empowerment* is an active level of community participation in which individuals, organizations, and communities gain mastery over their lives.

II. **Definition of Community Organization**
   A. Community organization is the process of developing competent community action systems and the technical tasks associated with their activities.
   B. Community organization describes the social structure of subsystems (agencies, organizations, mediating structures, sectors, etc.) within a community and the relationships among the subsystems.
   C. Community organization is a goal of community health nursing practice in which a community develops the ability to group and arrange its parts into a whole working system.
   D. Community organization is the process by which the community change agents empower individuals and aggregates to solve community problems and achieve community goals.

III. **Community Organization Models**
   A. *Rothman's Community Organization Typology* synthesizes community organization practice into models of social planning, social action, and locality development (community development).
      1. Social planning model
         a. Community decisions are based on fact gathering and rational decision making.
         b. Emphasis is placed on the task rather than the process.
         c. Roles of the community health nurse include facilitator, fact gatherer, analyst, and program implementor.
         d. Social planning is the practice model most universally supported by nursing theories.
      2. Social action model
         a. Community change is accomplished by polarization of the community around selected issues, followed by confrontation or conflict between people with opposing viewpoints.
         b. The major focus of social action is to transfer power to the aggregate.
         c. Roles of the community health nurse include community activist, agitator, and negotiator.

3. Community development model
   a. Community development emphasizes community involvement, self-direction, and self-help in determining and solving problems.
   b. The role of the community health nurse includes enabler and teacher of problem-solving skills. Because of this, community development is the preferred model for health promotion and protection.
   c. Community development is the community organization model considered by social science researchers to be most congruent with U.S. traditions, values, and beliefs. It is the most appropriate model for community nursing practice.
4. Community health development refers to community organizations that combine concepts, goals, and processes of community health and community development.
   a. Health-related needs are identified and health goals are established, met, and evaluated through community/professional partnerships.
   b. In this model, attributes of healthy communities include participation, capacity, and leadership.
   c. The primary roles of the nurse in this model are those of partner and leader.
B. Primary health care
1. Primary health care is community-based provision of essential health care (basic health care services) that is accessible to all members of the community.
2. Primary health care is practical, affordable, scientifically sound, and socially and culturally acceptable.
3. Primary health care is endorsed by the ANA as the preferred approach to community health nursing practice.
4. Primary health care is accomplished by a series of directed actions.
   a. Assessing the health status of individuals, families, and communities
   b. Prioritizing health needs
   c. Identifying resources and groups at risk
   d. Planning ways to meet priority health needs
   e. Implementing health promotion, disease prevention, case-finding, and curative services
   f. Promoting development of individual, family, and community competence to identify and meet their health needs

   g. Evaluating community health services and outcomes
C. Public health models and frameworks
1. The *Planned Approach to Community Health (PATCH)* is promoted by the Centers for Disease Control and Prevention. In PATCH, community members identify, prioritize, and act on aggregate health needs through community organization and decision making. Long-term solutions to health problems are encouraged by addressing the social, economic, environmental, and political precursors that contribute to problem development.
2. *Assessment Protocol for Excellence in Public Health (APEXPH)* uses community organization strategies to involve local communities in planning ways to meet *Healthy People* 2000 goals. APEXPH emphasizes building working partnerships between health departments and communities.
3. The *Health Cities Model* (health communities model) is an interaction model developed under WHO. It uses research to empower communities to take action to improve health.

IV. **Community Organization of Nursing Care of Aggregates**
A. Historic overview of nursing, community organization, and upstream thinking
1. Community organization has been incorporated into community health nursing practice since Florence Nightingale.
2. Community organization is implicit and explicit in current descriptions and standards of community health nursing practice.
3. The ANA and WHO identify community organization as a basic community health nursing skill.
B. Community organization strategies for nurses
1. Collaboration strategies
   a. Collaboration strategies are used when there is basic agreement on an issue or possible solution to a problem.
   b. The role of the nurse as change agent is enabler or facilitator.
   c. Collaboration strategies are applicable to the community development model.
2. Campaign strategies
   a. Campaign strategies can be used in situations in which people have different opinions about an issue or proposed solution, but the possibility of consensus exists.

b. The nurse is persuader and expert witness and uses epidemiological methods to gather data and identify major problems and groups at risk.

c. Campaign strategies fit the social planning model of change.

3. Contest strategies

a. Contest strategies are linked to social action approaches to change, including social action, nonviolence, and civil disobedience.

b. The nurse is an advocate, agitator, or contestant. He or she addresses inequities in health and health care by working within the system to bring about change or by assisting the client to force change.

c. Political mobilization and legislation are popular contrast strategies currently used in our government.

V. Application of the Nursing Process Through Community Organization

A. Social planning

1. The social planning model has been the model of community organization most frequently used by nurses in traditional community health agencies and organizations.

2. Advantages to this approach are speed and control of the planning process.

3. Disadvantages include lack of community or aggregate ownership and potential underuse or nonuse of nursing services.

B. Social action

1. In the social action model, the nurse is an advocate, agitator, activist, or negotiator on behalf of the aggregate.

2. This model is selected by nurses desiring political action or policy changes by governments and corporations.

3. A disadvantage is potential polarization around issues, which may interfere with mutual problem solving.

C. Community development

1. Within the community development model, assessment focuses on identification of perceived needs and potential resources of the community or aggregate.

2. Diagnoses are based on the community's priorities, and interventions are focused on community self-help, mobilization of resources, and integration of health care services.

3. Community development seeks two goals.

a. Active participation by individuals and aggregates in the community

b. Transfer of skills and knowledge needed to promote, protect, and restore the community's health to the individuals and aggregates.

c. Advantages of this approach include broad-based solutions to complex problems and community ownership of wealth.

d. A disadvantage is the length of time needed to effect change.

TEACHING STRATEGIES

1. Attend a city, county, or state government meeting in which health problems and health planning are discussed. Analyze which model (social planning, social action, or community development) is being used. What strategies are being used, and by whom? Are any nurses involved? What are their roles?

Community Health Education

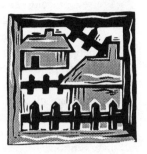

ANNOTATED LEARNING OBJECTIVES

1. Describe the aims of health education within the community.

Health education is "any combination of learning experiences designed to facilitate voluntary actions conducive to health that people can take on their own, individually or collectively, as citizens looking after their own health or as decision makers looking after the health of others and the common good of the community."

Health education is an important and integral aspect of professional community health nursing care, particularly in health promotion and disease prevention. Health education was identified as a nursing responsibility beginning with Florence Nightingale and is supported by the Nurse Practice Acts, the ANA, American Hospital Association, and the Joint Commission for the Accreditation of Healthcare Organizations (JCAHO).

The goal of health education is to help people understand health behavior and plan relevant interventions to promote health, prevent disease, and manage chronic illness. It is more than information dissemination. It includes interventions to guide people through the decision-making process about issues related to health.

2. Discuss the role of the nurse as health educator within a political and social context.

As health educators, it is important that community health nurses realize that cultural and social definitions of health differ. In addition, nurses must understand that individuals and communities must take responsibility for their own health.

Political efforts to improve the health of U.S. citizens were enhanced in the 1970s and 1980s with the passage of the National Consumer Health Information and Health Promotion Act and the establishment of the Bureau of Health Education. In addition, publication of *Healthy People* (1991) promulgated a number of goals and objectives to improve individual and community health. As a health educator, the community health nurse should disseminate health information to individuals, families, aggregates, and communities. The nurse should act as an advocate, counselor, and motivator and should work with groups to facilitate aggregate control over the aggregate's concerns and solutions.

3. Select a learning theory, and describe its application to an individual, family, or aggregate.

Learning theories developed from the field of psychology. A basic knowledge of various learning theories helps health care workers understand how individuals, families, and groups learn. There are several broad categories of learning theories, including behaviorist, cognitive, humanistic, and social learning.

Stimulus-Response Theory (behavior modification) is best applied to the individual because it is based on the concept of positive and negative reinforcement. It is important that the learner be actively involved.

Cognitive Field Theory is most applicable to the individual and small groups. Learning is individualized. It integrates bio/psycho/social and environmental factors. Interventions are directed at changing individual interpretations of reality (perceptions).

Adult Learning Theory, proposed by M. Knowles, can be used for education of individuals, families, or aggregates. Learning is independent, self-directed, and problem-oriented.

4. *Compare and contrast Freire's approach to health education with an individualistic health education model.*

Freire's Education Model applies the principles of social justice to the aggregate. Education is a tool to bring about empowerment. This model adds a sociopolitical dimension to learning. To apply Freire's model to health education, the problem(s) are defined by the client rather than by the provider, as in other models. Through conscientization (helping people discover and use unacknowledged power relationships to reduce distortions caused by domination), power is assumed by the community and changes are planned. After the problem has been identified by the community, the health educator contributes information to help plan appropriate interventions.

In contrast, the Health Belief Model (HBM) focuses on the individual. In the HBM, diseases are seen as negative influences on life, and preventive behaviors are directed at avoidance of illness and disease. The Health Belief Model can be used to direct learning toward changing individual perceptions of susceptibility and seriousness of a disease, barriers to change, and benefits of change. Educational efforts are directed at supplying information to change perceptions appropriately.

5. *Outline a systematic process for developing health education messages and programs.*

The National Cancer Institute uses six stages that are congruent with the nursing process, including a circular loop that provides for continuous assessment, feedback, and improvement. The model focuses on communication strategies in program planning and is applicable to individuals, families, and groups. This model consists of six stages:

Stage I:	Planning and Strategy Selection
Stage II:	Selecting Channels and Materials
Stage III:	Developing Materials and Pretesting
Stage IV:	Implementation
Stage V:	Assessing Effectiveness
Stage VI:	Feedback to Refine Program

6. *Identify resources of health education materials and describe their application for a given individual, family, or community as client.*

Sources for health education materials include professional organizations, hospitals, medical societies, volunteer and nonprofit organizations, commercial organizations, and government sources. Health education materials are useful tools that assist the nurse educator. It is important to select materials appropriate to the aggregate, considering culture, language, and literacy.

7. *Describe factors that enhance relevancy of health materials for an intended target group.*

All materials used in health education initiatives should be appropriate for the intended target audience. The nurse should ask questions such as:
- Is there a "fit" between the material and the target audience?
- Are the materials appealing?
- Is the message clear and understandable?
- Will the target audience identify and relate to the content, visuals, and written style?

Assessing the literacy level of the target audience is important. Many Americans have poor reading skills and difficulty with critical thinking. Individuals with very low literacy skills are at risk for poor health. Within Stage I, the nurse should use assessment skills to determine the reading level of the intended target audience. When developing health programs and materials for groups within the community, the nurse should ask a sample of potential target group members to review materials to ensure a match.

Within community sites, materials are collected, stored, and disseminated as needed. However, in many instances, pamphlets are distributed but not read or are skimmed so that they have little impact. It is important for nurses to evaluate health materials before they are disseminated to individuals, families, or the general public. Materials assessment should include format, layout, type, verbal content, visual content, and aesthetic quality. The nurse should also estimate the readability (grade level) of the printed text.

LECTURE OUTLINE

Health education refers to "any combination of learning experiences designed to facilitate voluntary actions conducive to health that people can take on their own, individually or collectively, as citizens looking after their own health or as decision makers looking after the health of others and the common good of the community."

I. **Health Education in the Community**
   A. Health education is an important and integral aspect of professional community health nursing care, particularly in the area of health promotion and disease prevention.
   B. Health education was identified as a nursing responsibility beginning with Florence Nightingale and is supported by the Nurse Practice Acts, the ANA, the American Hospital Association, and JCAHO.
   C. The goal of health education is to help people understand health behavior and plan relevant

interventions to promote health, prevent disease, and manage chronic illness.

D. Health education is more than information dissemination; it includes interventions to guide people through the decision-making process about issues related to health.

II. Learning Theories, Principles, and Health Education Models

A. Learning theories developed from the field of psychology and assist nurses as educators in understanding how individuals, families, and groups learn.

1. There are several broad categories of learning theories, including behaviorist, cognitive, humanistic and social learning.

    a. Cognitive theories (Lewin, Piaget) recognize the potential of the brain to think, feel, learn, and solve problems. The purpose of education is to train the brain to maximize those functions.

    b. Humanistic theories (Maslow) focus on facilitating the development of individuals toward their unique potential in a self-directing and holistic manner.

    c. Behavioral theories (Pavlov, Skinner) are based on the belief that learning is programmed through stimulus-response mechanisms that cause people to behave in a certain manner. Learning is based on condition or reinforcement.

    d. Social learning theories (Bandura) combine cognitive theories with behaviorism. These theories explain behavior and enhance learning through use of concepts of efficacy, outcome expectations, and incentives.

B. Knowles' assumptions about characteristics of adult learners

1. *Need to know*—Adults need to know why they need to learn.

2. *Self-concept*—Adults have a self-concept that has developed from dependence to independence; from others' direction to self-direction.

3. *Experience*—Adults have many life experiences from which to draw.

4. *Readiness to learn*—Developmental tasks and social roles affect readiness to learn. Timing learning experiences with developmental tasks is important.

5. *Orientation to learning*—Learning is present-oriented and "now"-based. Learning is directed to the immediate need and is problem-centered.

6. *Motivation*—Internal drives and factors (self-esteem, life goals, responsibility) are powerful motivators.

C. Health education models form a theoretical basis for planning community nursing interventions. Theoretical frameworks offer nurses a blueprint for interventions that promote learning and provide them with an organized approach to explaining relationships of concepts.

1. Models of individual behavior

    a. The *health belief model (HBM)* is based on social psychology and was developed to help understand why people did not participate in health education programs to prevent or detect disease. The HBM addresses factors that promote health-enhancing behaviors, rather than the inhibiting factors. Dimensions considered by the HBM include perceived susceptibility, severity, benefits, and barriers; self-efficacy; demographics; and "cues to action." The HBM focuses on individual, rather than socio/environmental, determinants of behavior.

    b. The *health promotion model* modified concepts of the HBM and focused on predicting behaviors particularly with regard to health promotion. Additional factors were added (perceived control, perceived importance of health, and interpersonal influence).

2. Model of health education empowerment

    a. Individual models fail to account fully for the complex relationships between social, structural, and physical factors in the environment (unemployment, lack of social support systems, inaccessible health services, and racism).

    b. Citizen participation is key for effective and successful health promotion programs.

    c. Reconceptualizing health beyond the individual to the group is based on empowerment and community participation.

        1) Important concepts in empowering health education and social justice include neighborhood as base, development of comprehensive education strategies and programming, and community empowerment.

        2) At the core of empowerment is information, communication, and health

education that involves individuals, families, and groups in learning.

3) Nurses can use empowerment strategies to help people develop skills in problem solving, networking, negotiating, lobbying, and information seeking to enhance heath.

D. Community empowerment

1. Creating change at the community level requires the nurse to be knowledgeable about key concepts of community organization.

2. The nurse should help the community identify common goals, develop strategies, and mobilize resources to increase community empowerment.

3. Citizens may need assistance in learning to assume responsibility for decision making about their own health and the health of the community.

4. Power is shifted away from health providers toward community members to address health priorities. Collaboration and cooperation can help ensure that community needs are met.

III. **The Nurse's Role in Health Education**

A. At the core of health education is a therapeutic relationship that develops between the nurse and individuals, families, and the community.

B. Nurses can move ideas into action, offer interventions, identify resources, and facilitate group empowerment.

IV. **Putting Models and Theories into Action—** Using a systematic approach to health education is essential for community health nurses. The National Cancer Institute uses a six-stage model of a systemic approach, similar to the nursing process, with a circular loop that provides for continuous assessment, feedback, and improvement. The model focuses on communication strategies in program planning and is applicable to individuals, families, and groups.

A. Stage I: Planning and Strategy Selection—This stage focuses on understanding the learning needs of the target audience and targeting the program or message to the audience. The needs of the target audience are determined, and an open dialogue is created.

1. Questions to ask

a. Who is the target audience?

b. What are goals and objectives?

c. What is the health issue of interest?

2. Collaborative actions to take

a. Review available data from health statistics, libraries, newspapers, and community leaders

b. Obtain new data from interviews or focus groups

c. Determine the group's needs and perception of health problems

d. Identify related issues

e. Identify existing gaps of health knowledge

f. Write goals and objectives

g. Assess resources

B. Stage II: Selecting Channels and Materials— *Channel* refers to how the nurse will reach target groups. *Format* refers to how the message will be communicated. *Materials/media* are tools of a program.

1. Questions to ask

a. What channels are best?

b. What formats should be used?

c. Are there existing resources?

2. Collaborative actions to take

a. Identify messages and materials to be used

b. Decide whether to use existing materials or create new ones

c. Select channels and formats

C. Stage III: Developing Materials and Pretesting— Different types of communication concepts may be developed in the first stages and can be tested with the target audience for feedback.

1. Questions to ask

a. How can the message be presented?

b. How will the target audience react to the message?

c. Will the audience understand, accept, and use the message?

d. What changes might improve the message?

2. Collaborative actions to take

a. Develop relevant materials with the target audience

b. Pretest materials and messages and obtain feedback from the audience.

D. Stage IV: Implementation—In this stage, the health education message and programs are introduced to the target audience and components are reviewed and revised.

1. Questions to ask

a. Are the message and program getting to the target audience?

b. Do any channels need to be altered?

c. What are the strengths of the health program?

      d. What changes would enhance effective-
         ness?
   2. Collaborative actions to take
      a. Work with community organizations,
         businesses, and other health agencies to
         enhance effectiveness
      b. Monitor progress
      c. Establish evaluation measures

E. Stage V: Assessing Effectiveness—The program and health message should be analyzed
for effectiveness using the mechanism identified in Stage I. Process and summative
evaluation, as well as outcome evaluation, may
be used.
   1. Questions to ask
      a. Were objectives met?
      b. What was the impact?
      c. How well did each step work?
      d. Were changes realized as a result of the
         program?
   2. Collaborative actions to take include con-
      ducting process and outcome evaluations.

F. Stage VI: Feedback to Refine Program—The
information gained from the audience, the
channels of communication, and the program's
intended effects can be used to prepare for a
new cycle of development. Information should
be used to validate program strengths and
allow for modifications.
   1. Questions to ask
      a. What was learned?
      b. What can be improved on?
      c. What worked well, and what did not?
      d. Are the goals and objectives relevant?
      e. What modifications can be made to
         strengthen the health education activity?
   2. Collaborative actions to take
      a. Reassess goals and objectives
      b. Revise as needed
      c. Modify strategies or activities that did
         not succeed
      d. Summarize the health education pro-
         gram in an evaluation report
      e. Provide justification for continuing the
         program or ending it.

V. **Health Education Resources**—Health education
materials and resources are available from local,
state, and national organizations and agencies.
Nurses can help individuals, families, and groups
gain access to needed materials, services, or equipment by being knowledgeable about available
resources.

A. Information and materials for health education
are available from a number of sources. (The

text presents a comprehensive list of health
education resources.)
   1. Local and regional hospitals, libraries, and
      businesses
   2. Federal, state, and local governments
   3. Community-based organizations
   4. Colleges and universities
   5. Professional organizations
   6. Commercial organizations
   7. Voluntary agencies

B. The nurse should assess the relevancy of health
materials.
   1. All materials used in health education ini-
      tiatives should be appropriate for the target
      audience.
   2. The nurse should ask the following questions.
      a. Is there a "fit" between the material and
         the target audience?
      b. Are the materials appealing?
      c. Is the message clear and understand-
         able?
      d. Will the target audience identify and
         relate to the content, visuals, and writ-
         ten style?

C. Assessing the literacy level of the target audience is important.
   1. Many Americans have poor reading skills
      and have difficulty with critical thinking.
   2. Individuals with very low literacy skills are
      at risk for poor health.
   3. Within Stage I, the nurse should use assess-
      ment skills to determine the reading level
      of the intended target audience.
   4. When developing health programs and
      materials for groups within the community,
      the nurse should ask a sample of potential
      target group members to review the mate-
      rials to ensure a match.

D. The nurse should try to evaluate how the materials will be received by the community.
   1. Within community sites, materials are often
      collected, stored, and disseminated as
      needed. However, in many instances, pam-
      phlets are distributed but not read or are
      only skimmed, so they have little impact.
   2. It is important for the nurse to evaluate
      health materials before they are dissemi-
      nated to individuals, families, or the general
      public.
   3. Material assessment should include format,
      layout, type, verbal content, visual content,
      and aesthetic quality.
   4. The nurse should estimate the readability
      (grade level) of the printed text.

TEACHING STRATEGIES

1. Identify a community health problem for which a health education program would be appropriate (e.g., teenage pregnancy, teenage gangs, violence, driving under the influence of alcohol, or failure to immunize infants). Gather information from the media (newspapers, television, radio, magazines) related to the problem. What messages are observed? What strategies have been taken by the community to deal with the problem? How has the community been involved in identifying the problem and potential solutions?

2. Collect health education materials (pamphlets, booklets, brochures, posters) on a variety of topics and from a number of sources. Divide the class into groups of 3–4 students and have them analyze the materials using the criteria described in the chapter. Have each group report briefly on the materials to the class.

3. Assign each student one of the health educational materials discussed above. Have students assess the materials using the "Rapid Estimate of Adult Literacy in Medicine" (REALM) tool (Figure 8-3) and present findings to the class.

Policy, Politics, Legislation, and Public Health Nursing

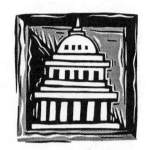

ANNOTATED LEARNING OBJECTIVES

1. Describe the role nurses have played in influencing the public's health through policy development.

Beginning with Florence Nightingale in the mid-1960s, nurses have influenced public policy, both individually and collectively, at the local, state, federal, and international levels.

An example of individual effort is Nightingale's use of her personal resources and influential family to provide care to British soldiers in the Crimean war. Another example is nursing student Carrie Long, who worked to improve the living conditions for a group of families in south Texas by enlisting assistance from area health departments, a local judge, and others.

Nursing's Agenda for Healthcare Reform is an example of a recent collective effort by nurses to address issues relating to the health care delivery system. In addition, a number of nurses were involved in the health care reform task force headed by Hillary Clinton in the early 1990s.

2. Analyze public policy as the critical basis for protecting the public's health.

Public policy directs activities, sets goals, and influences politics. Health care policy is integral to ensure the health and well-being of citizens. Much of the protection of the public's health is achieved through policy setting at the local, county, state, federal, and international levels.

3. Identify the legislative process involved in establishing state or federal health policy.

A multistep process is used to establish health policy. Initially, a problem must be defined, and the problem must become an item on the legislative agenda. Supporters of the policy then obtain a

commitment of resources (funding) by passing legislation. A schedule is formed for implementing the law into a program. Finally, a formal design for evaluation is set up.

4. Identify the political processes that influence health policy development.

Authority for the protection of the public's health is largely vested in the states. Each state establishes policies or standards for goods and services that affect the health of its citizens. The federal government is involved in matters involving interstate commerce and the "general welfare" of citizens.

Decisions that affect public health are made at each governmental branch. The legislative branch enacts laws. The executive branch and regulatory agencies administer and enforce the laws. The judicial branch provides protection against professional malpractice, fraud, and abuse.

5. Discuss political activities through which nurses can affect the health policies of their community and country.

Nurses can affect health policy through a variety of activities. For example, a nurse may campaign for a political candidate with whom the nurse shares similar viewpoints. The nurse may act as a lobbyist to influence policy makers or become involved in political action committees, professional associations, and coalitions to help influence health policy.

LECTURE OUTLINE

I. **Nurses Who Made a Difference**

    A. *Florence Nightingale*—When recruited in the 1850s to help the British Army in the Crimean war, Nightingale took 38 nurses to care for the soldiers. When the nurses arrived, the mortality rate for injured soldiers was 60%; at the end of the war it was slightly over 1%. One of the contributing factors to Nightingale's success was her ability to gain and use power.

B. *Carrie Long*—In the 1980s, Carrie Long was a nursing student in Monaco, Texas, when she discovered numerous sanitation problems in a housing development predominantly inhabited by low-income Hispanic families. She performed a community assessment, including review of relevant Texas state laws and morbidity/mortality statistics. Using this information, she was able to influence interventions at the county level on behalf of the Hispanic families.

II. **Nurses: Agents of Change**

A. The government and the public recognize nurses as necessary and valued resources.

B. Nurses are professionals whose knowledge, skill, and concern are used to promote society's well-being.

C. Because they are interpreters of the health care system to the public, public health nurses in particular are profoundly influenced by government interventions. Therefore, public health nurses must know how to participate in the political process.

III. **Public Policy: Blueprint for Governance**—Public policy articulates the guiding principles of collective endeavors, establishes direction, and sets goals.

A. Policy formulation in an "ideal world"

1. Ideally, health care policy would be created by groups that determine what should be done on the basis of valid data.

2. Whether a policy is advocated or adopted would depend on the degree to which a group or society might benefit without harm or detriment to subgroups.

3. Group need and group demand would be the strongest determinants of health policy.

4. There would be equitable distribution of services and the assurance that the appropriate care would be given to the right people at the right time for a reasonable cost.

B. Policy formulation in the "real world"

1. In reality, health care policy is the product of a continuous interactive process in which "interested" professionals, citizens, institutions, and other groups compete with each other for the attention of various branches of the government.

2. Health policy usually evolves slowly as an accumulation of many small decisions.

C. Steps in policy formation

1. Define the problem.

2. Get the problem into the legislative agenda.

3. Obtain commitment of resources (funding) by passing legislation.

4. Formulate a schedule for implementing the law into a program.

5. Design an evaluation process.

D. Policy analysis

1. Analysis of health policy is an objective process that identifies the sources and consequences of decisions in the context of the factors that influence them.

2. Health policy analysis identifies those who benefit and those who experience a loss as the result of a policy.

IV. **Health Care Reform and the Nursing Agenda**

A. *Nursing's Agenda for Healthcare Reform* was developed collaboratively by the ANA and the NLN to address inadequacies and inequality in the American health care delivery system. The agenda helped promote understanding of nursing and its contributions to health care.

B. Nurses were an integral part of Hillary Rodham Clinton's task force for health care reform. Their efforts failed to change national policy due to a number of factors, primarily the complexity of the plan and opposition from the insurance industry and provider groups.

V. **Government: The Hallmark of Civilization**

A. Government is the exercise of political authority, direction, and restraint over the actions of inhabitants of communities, societies, or states. It is crucial to human interdependence and necessary for cooperative action.

B. Government regulates conditions beyond the control of individuals.

C. The U.S. Constitution declares a responsibility to "promote the general welfare," which has been interpreted to include health matters.

VI. **Government Authority for the Protection of the Public's Health**

A. The authority for the protection of the public's health is largely vested in the states; therefore, the state is a critical arena for political action.

B. Each state establishes policies or standards for goods and services that affect the health of its citizens.

C. The federal government oversees matters involving interstate commerce and "general welfare" cases. Conformance by states to federal program standards is voluntary, but revenue is withheld from the states if they do not comply.

VII. Balance of Powers: Safeguard of Government— Decisions affecting the public's health are made at each governmental branch.
  A. The legislative branch enacts the statutory laws that are the basis for governance.
  B. Through regulatory agencies, the executive branch administers and enforces the laws enacted by the legislative branch. The regulatory agencies define implementation of the statutes through rules and regulations.
  C. The judiciary branch provides protection against oppressive governance, professional malpractice, and abuse.

VIII. Politics in Action—The Legislative Process
  A. The legislative process is a mode of intervention on behalf of the public.
  B. When passing a bill, the opposition has the advantage.
  C. To become law, an idea must overcome several hurdles.
    1. A concept is drafted into legislative language and becomes a bill.
    2. The bill must pass through one or more committees and be approved by both houses of the legislature.
    3. The bill is then approved (or vetoed) by the chief executive.

IX. The Individual Nurse's Role in Politics
  A. Lobbying
    1. A lobbyist is a person who represents special interests, typically to legislators.
    2. Legislators rely on lobbyists for education on issues.
    3. Influencing lawmakers to pass effective health legislation requires the participation of individual nurses as well as organizations.
    4. To lobby effectively, the nurse must first establish herself as a concerned constituent and a credible source of information on health issues.
  B. Campaigning
    1. Helping someone win an election is one way to gain influence.
    2. Campaign activities can be in the form of contributions or voluntary activities such as setting up social gatherings, stuffing envelopes, or answering telephones.

X. The Collective Power of Nurses—In the United States, there are more than 2 million nurses—the largest single discipline in health care. Therefore, when nurses unite, they have enormous power. There are several ways to exert that power.

  A. Professional associations
    1. Collective action by nursing and health care organizations such as ANA and APHA helps meet identified goals. These associations monitor legislative activity related to health issues and distribute information to their membership.
    2. The ANA and APHA have full-time staff lobbyists who work with Congress, but the greatest influence on elected officials is generally exerted when they receive sufficiently high numbers of communications (letters and telephone calls) from individual constituents.
  B. Political action committees (PACs)
    1. Political action committees are nonpartisan entities that promote the election of candidates believed to be sympathetic to their interests.
    2. PACs are established by professional associations and business and labor groups that contribute financially to campaigns.
  C. Coalitions
    1. A coalition is formed when two or more groups join to maximize resources for the purpose of achieving a common goal.
    2. Coalitions of health care providers often work together on issues that may cross several disciplines, such as family violence, women's health, substance abuse, and AIDS.

XI. Nursing and the Health of the Nation—A Social Contract
  A. As a profession, nursing derives its status from a contract with society to provide essential services under conditions of altruism.
  B. Nurses serve the healthy and the sick, and they should use their influence to promote wellness through public policy.
  C. Both nurses and the public should constantly be attuned to opportunities to promote the appointment or election of nurses to policy-making positions.

TEACHING STRATEGIES

  1. Contact groups or organizations that work to influence public health issues from a variety of viewpoints (women's groups, child protection groups, NOW, National Right to Life, MADD, etc.). Obtain literature from these organizations regarding the purpose of the group and methods they use to influence public policy. Divide the class into groups

and have them debate pro/con issues from a political perspective.

2. Early in the semester, have the class choose one or two issues or bills pending in the state legislature. Have students attempt to affect the legislative process by writing letters to people in congress, making telephone calls, or writing letters to the editor of the local paper. Encourage students to follow the issue or bill throughout the semester for progress.

3. Identify current issues that affect health and health care delivery, such as changes in Medicaid or Medicare, speed limit increases, nonsmoking legislation, or gun control. Have students outline the existing policy and trace the formulation of the policy in the literature.

4. Obtain a copy of *Nursing's Agenda for Healthcare Reform*. Discuss which components have been implemented and which have not. What factors have hindered the implementation? What policy changes must be made to accomplish the suggested changes? How can nurses join together to help make these changes?

CHAPTER 10

Child and Adolescent Health

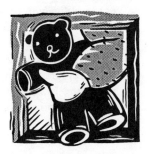

ANNOTATED LEARNING OBJECTIVES

1. Identify the major indicators of child and adolescent health status.

The major indicators of child and adolescent health status are infant mortality (due to low birth weight, lack of prenatal care, substance abuse by the mother, or socioeconomic status); accidental injuries; violence; and "new morbidities of youth" (teenage pregnancy, STDs, AIDS, and substance abuse.

2. Describe how socioeconomic circumstances influence child and adolescent health.

Poverty is associated with poor health status. Poverty is often associated with single-parent households (most commonly single women). Teen pregnancy, poor education, low income, and lack of social support contribute to poor health status. Poor children are at risk of death from unintended injuries, child abuse, SIDS, lead poisoning, and infectious diseases. They are also less likely to be immunized. Adolescents living in poverty are at risk for homicide, teen pregnancy, substance abuse, and gang involvement.

3. Discuss the individual and societal costs of poor child health status.

Lack of adequate prenatal care contributes greatly to an increased incidence of low-birthweight infants. Prenatal care can save more than three dollars for every dollar spent in direct medical costs. In addition, complications of prematurity include sensory deficiencies, decreased mental capacity, and mental retardation, all resulting in long-term educational and societal consequences.

Lead poisoning is one of the leading preventable causes of mental retardation. It affects approximately one in six children in the United States. Lead poisoning is also associated with behavior problems and poor school performance, which contribute to additional problems.

Drug abuse and delinquency prevention and treatment for addicted mothers can save thousands of dollars in medical care, foster care, and special education for drug-exposed babies. Prevention of adolescent pregnancy can reduce welfare dependency, low birth weight, infant mortality, and the rate at which adolescents drop out of school.

4. Discuss public programs targeted to children's health.

Medicaid is a combined federal/state program to provide health care services to the poor. Recently, eligibility for pregnant women, infants, and children has been increased to improve infant mortality.

The *Early and Periodic Screening, Diagnosis, and Treatment (EPSDT)* program provides health, development, and nutritional screening; physical examinations; immunizations; vision and hearing screening; dental services; and some laboratory tests for eligible children.

The *Maternal and Child Health Block Grant* is a federally funded program to provide health care to pregnant women and children.

The *Community and Migrant Health Centers Program* provides primary health care to 6 million low-income people (about one third of whom are children).

National Health Service Corps is a federal program that provides primary health care services in underserved rural or urban areas.

Supplemental Food Program for Women, Infants, and Children (WIC) provides food and nutrition education to low-income pregnant and breastfeeding mothers and their children under the age of 5.

Head Start is a federally funded, comprehensive early childhood program that provides educational opportunities, medical care, dental care, and nutritional and social services for low-income children ages 3–5.

5. *Apply knowledge of child health needs in planning appropriate, comprehensive care to children at the individual, family, and community levels.*

The community health nurse should combine knowledge of major indicators of child health, social factors that contribute to declining health status, and public programs designed to address problems of plan care. Efforts should encompass all levels of prevention (primary, secondary, tertiary) and should address needs of the individual, family, and community.

LECTURE OUTLINE

I. **Indicators of Child and Adolescent Health Status**
   A. Pregnancy and infancy
      1. Infant mortality
         a. Infant mortality is often seen as a marker of the health and welfare of an entire community or society.
         b. In 1992, the United States ranked 24th in infant mortality among industrialized nations.
         c. Black infants have, by far, the highest infant mortality rate in the country.
         d. The leading causes of neonatal death are congenital anomalies, prematurity, and effects of maternal complications.
      2. Low birthweight
         a. Low-birthweight (infants born weighing less than 5.5 pounds) is the overall leading cause of infant mortality.
         b. Nearly 300,000 low-birthweight babies (about 7% of the total) are born each year in the United States, with twice as many black low-birthweight infants as white.
         c. Associated problems include mental disabilities, blindness, deafness, learning disabilities, and mental retardation.
         d. Risk factors associated with low birthweight include lack of prenatal care, maternal smoking, alcohol and drug use, and low socioeconomic status.
      3. Lack of prenatal care
         a. Babies born to women with no prenatal care are three times as likely to be born with low birthweight.
         b. One fourth of all pregnant women in the United States fail to receive prenatal care beginning in the first trimester.
         c. Thorough prenatal care can hlep spot threats to successful pregnancy, provide health education and counseling, and direct low-income women to obtain social services such as WIC, food stamps, and treatment for substance abuse.
         d. Women who are poor, unmarried, young, and in the minority are less likely to receive prenatal care.
         e. Barriers to receiving timely prenatal care include financial barriers, lack of insurance, high deductibles and copayments, inadequate supply of providers, lack of coordinated services, insensitive cultural conditions, personal attitudes, lifestyle conditions, and knowledge deficit regarding the need for prenatal care.
      4. Prenatal substance use—Substance (illegal drugs, alcohol, cigarettes) use during pregnancy is linked with poor outcomes.
         a. Illegal drug use—Five percent of women use illegal drugs while pregnant (1992). The most serious consequence is the prenatal transmission of STDs, particularly HIV.
         b. Smoking—Smoking during pregnancy is the most common source of prenatal exposure to drugs. It is associated with low-birthweight infants, SIDS, and childhood asthma.
   B. Childhood
      1. Accidental injuries
         a. After the first year, accidental injury (motor vehicle injury, drowning, suffocation, and burning) is the leading cause of death of children.
         b. Motor vehicle accidents involving pedestrians or bicycles are a major cause of child deaths.
      2. Lead poisoning
         a. Lead poisoning is a preventable cause of death, mental retardation, cognitive and behavioral problems, and other disabilities in children.
         b. In the United States, one out of every six children under the age of 6 has blood levels that are dangerously high, making lead poisoning the most prevalent disease of environmental origin among U.S. children.

3. Child abuse and neglect
   a. More than 3 million children were reportedly abused or neglected in 1994, and approximately 1,000 U.S. children die each year from abuse and neglect.
   b. Most cases involve children under the age of 5.
   c. Dominant characteristics of abusive parents are a history of substance abuse and having been abused themselves as children.
C. Adolescence
   1. Violence
      a. Beginning in adolescence, suicide and homicide are major causes of death.
      b. Homicide is the second leading cause of death for people aged 15–24 and the leading cause of death for black males.
      c. Violence affects minorities disproportionately. Reasons include social factors of unemployment; poverty; gang exposure; easy availability of handguns; witnessing violence in the home, media and community; and being a victim of child abuse.
   2. Teenage pregnancy
      a. Approximately 1 million girls become pregnant each year.
      b. Teenage pregnancy poses health risks to the baby, including death, prematurity, low birth weight, and neglect.
   3. Sexually transmitted diseases
      a. Teenagers have the highest rates of STDs among heterosexuals of all age groups.
      b. Women are particularly at risk for complications associated with STDs.
      c. Chlamydia and gonorrhea are the most common STDs.
   4. Substance abuse
      a. Approximately one third of adolescents are thought to drink alcohol in excess, and one fourth have reported that they have used an illicit drug.
      b. Tobacco use is prevalent among adolescents, and nearly all initial uses of tobacco occur before graduation from high school.

II. **Social Factors Affecting Child Health**—Children living in poor households, those from single-parent families, those from minority cultures, and those without health insurance coverage are more likely to suffer from health problems.
A. Poverty

1. In 1993, approximately 23% of children under age 6 lived in poverty.
2. Children comprise 40% of the poor.
3. Deaths from unintended injuries, child abuse, SIDS, and infectious diseases are more common in this group.
B. Single-parent households
   1. Children in households headed by single women are much more likely to live in poverty.
   2. Teenage pregnancy, poor education, low income, and lack of social support contribute to poor health in the children.
C. Adolescence
   1. Adolescence is a period of growing independence and risk-taking behaviors. During this time, the responsibility for health is moving from the parent to the teen.
   2. Obstacles for health-seeking behaviors
      a. Attitudinal or behavioral factors
      b. Concerns over confidentiality
      c. Embarrassment and unwillingness to seek help for sensitive problems (matters dealing with sexual health, mental health, or substance abuse)

III. **Costs to Society of Poor Health Among Children**—For no other age group is prevention of health problems more significant or cost effective. Primary health care and early intervention for children and families can help prevent costly problems.
A. Prenatal care
   1. Prenatal care can save hundreds of thousands of dollars by preventing conditions, such as low birthweight, that require expensive medical treatment after an infant has been born.
   2. It has been estimated that for every dollar spent on prenatal care for high-risk women, more than three dollars can be saved on the cost of providing direct medical care during the first year of an infant's life.
B. Lead poisoning
   1. There is no cure for lead poisoning; therefore, the most cost-effective treatment is prevention.
   2. Removal of the sources of lead in the environment is expensive, but not as expensive as the long-term consequences of lead poisoning.
C. Adolescent pregnancy and parenting—preventing pregnancy among school-age mothers can reduce welfare dependency, low birth weight, infant mortality, and the rate at which adolescents drop out of school.

IV. Public Health Programs Targeted to Children

A. Medicaid

1. The ability of poor children to obtain health care services has improved since the introduction of Medicaid and the Early and Periodic Screening, Diagnosis, and Treatment (EPSDT) program.

2. Recently, Medicaid eligibility for pregnant women, infants, and children has been increased in an effort to improve the nation's infant mortality rate and children's health status.

3. EPSDT services include health, developmental, and nutritional screening; physical examinations; immunizations; vision ahd hearing screening; certain laboratory tests; and dental services.

4. Barriers that prohibit some children from receiving Medicaid services

   a. Lengthy application forms and eligibility determination processes

   b. The stigma of welfare that is associated with Medicaid

   c. Increasing numbers of physicians unwilling to take Medicaid patients

   d. Unfriendly, overcrowded, uncomfortable waiting rooms and public clinics

B. Direct health and care delivery programs

1. Maternal and Child Health Block Grant

   a. This is a federally funded program in which designated funds are allocated to the states.

   b. The states add their own funds and provide funds to local public health clinics to deliver health care to pregnant women and children.

2. Community and Migrant Health Centers Program

   a. This program began in 1965.

   b. It currently operates more than 2000 clinics to provide comprehensive primary health care to 6 million low-income people.

3. National Health Service Corps

   a. This is a federal program through which children receive primary health care services.

   b. The NHSC sends physicians, nurses, and other health care providers to underserved areas of the country. The program assists students with medical, nursing, and other training in return for a certain number of years of service in an underserved area.

4. Special Supplemental Food Program for Women, Infants, and Children (WIC)

   a. WIC provides nutritious foods and nutrition education to low-income pregnant and breastfeeding mothers and their children under the age of 5.

   b. Established in 1972, WIC has been successful, popular, and cost-effective.

   c. Despite its success, all those eligible for WIC cannot be enrolled due to funding limitations.

5. Head Start

   a. Head Start is a federally funded comprehensive early childhood program for low-income children ages 3–5.

   b. Head Start provides educational opportunities for children, as well as medical, dental, mental health, nutritional, and social services.

   c. In 1993, approximately 36% of eligible children were enrolled in Head Start.

V. Strategies to Improve Child Heath

A. Parents' role

1. Before and during pregnancy, a mother must develop healthy behaviors, including proper nutrition and avoidance of smoking, alcohol, drugs, and other behaviors that could harm her fetus.

2. Parents must give their children proper nutrition and ensure that they are immunized and receive needed health care services and acquire healthful lifestyles.

3. They should also ensure that their children have a safe environment at home, in the neighborhood, and at school.

B. Community's role

1. Communities should help create safe neighborhoods; support the development of community-based health programs; and promote community health education campaigns concerning prenatal care, smoking, nutrition, and other health topics.

2. Communities should encourage "one-stop shopping" for health and health-related services needed by children and families.

C. Employers' role

1. An employer can make health care more accessible to families with children by offering affordable health insurance that covers employees and dependents.

2. Employers can provide for adequate sick and family leave and sponsor opportunities for employees to learn about healthy diets, pregnancies, and ways to decrease stress.

3. Businesses can offer on-site child care.
D. Government's role
   1. Despite the number of programs and funds committed to children's health, many children do not receive the services they need.
   2. Effective programs for underserved populations should be expanded
   3. Collaborative efforts by nurses, physicians, social workers, and caseworkers should be encouraged.
E. Community health nurses' role
   1. It is the community health nurse's responsibility to advocate improved individual and community responses to the needs of children; to participate in publicly funded programs; and to network with other professionals to improve collaboration and coordination of services.
   2. An important role of the community health nurse is to help link community health services with the school system.

TEACHING STRATEGIES

1. Divide the class into groups of three or four and have each group research a different community service provider that works with children, adolescents, or pregnant women in the area. For example, one group can identify the availability of immunizations for low-income families; another group can contact WIC to explore the process for enrolling in the program; another group can contact Medicaid and obtain information about enrolling. Have each group present their findings to the class.

2. Obtain infant mortality statistics on the local community. Compare rates with those of other communities within the state and the nation. Discuss similarities and differences. Attempt to explain why differences exist.

3. Invite a case worker from area child protective services to speak to the class about child abuse. Encourage the speaker to include information on possible indicators of child abuse and the process of reporting.

Women's Health

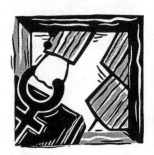

ANNOTATED LEARNING OBJECTIVES

1. Discuss the incidence and prevalence of gender-specific health problems.

Although women use health services at a higher rate than men, they have significantly higher life expectancies. Men have higher rates of heart disease than women (prior to menopause) and higher rates of death from lung cancer, although women's rates are increasing dramatically. Women have higher rates of diabetes, hypertension, and arthritis. In addition, women have more surgeries, more hospitalizations for mental illness, more hospitalizations for physical problems, and higher rates of disability than men.

2. Determine the major indicators of women's health.

Major indicators of women's health include life expectancy, mortality, morbidity, and other factors such as education, health behavior, and health care access.

3. Relate the impact of poverty on the health of women.

Poor and minority women have less access to health care than most women. In general, they also have shorter life spans, greater maternal mortality rates, shorter survival rates for cancer, and higher levels of stress related to family configuration (single parenting).

4. Identify barriers to adequate health care for women.

Barriers to health care for women include poverty, lack of access to care, lack of knowledge about health problems and health threats, and lack of knowledge about the availability of social services and health care providers.

5. Discuss the impact of public policy on the health of women.

Medicaid and Medicare have improved access and delivery of health care to eligible women. The Public Health Service Act provides health services, research, and information dissemination for women's health concerns. The Civil Rights Act prohibits discrimination against pregnant women and sexual harassment in the workplace. The Occupational Safety and Health Act works to ensure worksite safety for all citizens.

6. Apply the nursing process to women's health concerns in the community.

Assessment of women's health needs should be comprehensive and should include physical, psychological, social, and spiritual areas. Socioeconomic status, education, spouse and family support, and social services should be addressed. Analysis and diagnosis should be based on assessment data and should include a review of the available health services.

Planning should be collaborative in nature when possible, including care providers from other disciplines such as social services. Strategies should be formulated to address all levels of prevention (primary, secondary, tertiary).

Interventions should be directed at the individual, family, aggregate, or community level as applicable. Efforts to address social and community issues that contribute to the problem should be included.

Evaluation should be based on outcomes and identified goals.

7. Discuss reproductive health in relationship to the workplace.

Reproductive risks associated with exposure to occupational health hazards include altered fertility, spontaneous abortion, congenital malformations, intrauterine growth retardation, and fetal death. The Occupational Safety and Health Act was enacted in 1970 to promote healthy worksites. Occupational health nurses must be aware of hazards at their workplaces. They should routinely collect data on potential risk factors in the relevant occupational environment.

8. *Examine prominent health problems among women of all age groups (from adolescent to old age).*

Adolescent women are at risk for pregnancy and related problems, STDs, dysmenorrhea, and nutritional deficiencies. Young women have health concerns related to fertility, infertility and pregnancy, dysmenorrhea, and depression. Middle-aged women have an increasing potential for malignancies (particularly of the breast, lung, and reproductive tract), heart disease, diabetes, hypertension, arthritis, and problems associated with menopause. Older women are at risk for accidents, osteoporosis, cerebrovascular disease, and cancers of the breast and reproductive system.

9. *Discuss primary, secondary and tertiary prevention stages as they relate to women's health.*

Primary prevention strategies for women's health include ensuring proper nutrition throughout the life span, family planning and use of contraception, prevention of STDs and AIDS, prevention of osteoporosis, and stress reduction.

Secondary prevention includes screening for cancer of the cervix (through pap tests), breast self-examination (BSE), mammography, pregnancy testing, AIDS testing, and routine gynecological exams.

Tertiary prevention includes care for high-risk pregnancies; treatment of AIDS, cancer, and other chronic illnesses; and treatment of mental illnesses such as depression.

10. *State the necessity for increased research efforts focused on women's health issues and their needs.*

Although women are the major users of health care in the United States, little research has been conducted to provide information for prediction, explanation, or description of phenomena affecting the health of women. Medical treatment is generally based on research in which the subjects were exclusively male. Research directed specifically at women's health needs is being instituted. Current efforts focus on topics such as osteoporosis, health promotion and education, menopause, dysmenorrhea, contraception, and domestic violence.

LECTURE OUTLINE

I. **Major Indicators of Health**
   A. Life expectancy—The female sex has the advantage in longevity in most countries.
      1. Males born in 1992 have a life expectancy of 72.3 years, compared with 79.0 years for females.
      2. Black females born in 1992 can expect to live 75.9 years, and white females 79.7 years.
   B. Mortality
      1. Leading causes of death
         a. The leading cause of death for both men and women is heart disease, although the death rate for heart disease has declined considerably in the last 30 years. Cardiovascular diseases account for 51.8% of deaths among females in the United States.
         b. Accidents are the leading cause of death for young women ages 15 to 24.
         c. Malignant neoplasm is the leading cause of death in women ages 25 to 64.
      2. Maternal mortality
         a. Since the 1950s, maternal mortality has declined steadily in the United States due to improved prenatal care, early detection of maternal risk, improved anesthesia, and antibiotics.
         b. Major risk factors for maternal deaths include inadequate access to prenatal care, poor nutrition, and substandard living conditions.
         c. The leading cause of maternal mortality is pulmonary embolism, followed by hypertensive disorders, ectopic pregnancy, stroke, and anesthesia.
         d. Ectopic pregnancy is the leading cause of maternal deaths during the first trimester. Teenagers, particularly nonwhite, are at risk for ectopic pregnancy.
      3. Malignant neoplasms
         a. Cancer death rates among women have increased steadily in the last 35 years.
         b. Over the last 30 years, lung cancer has increased by 450% in women, but only by 96% in men.
         c. In 1987, lung cancer surpassed breast cancer as the leading cause of cancer death in women.
         d. Early diagnosis and prompt treatment are major factors in surviving many types of cancer. Five-year survival rates

vary according to the type of cancer and its stage at diagnosis.

    e. Risk reduction strategies such as not smoking, improving nutrition, and limiting alcohol can help decrease cancer rates.

4. Cardiovascular disease and diabetes mellitus

    a. In the United States, more people die from cardiovascular disease than from any other condition.

    b. Rates of death from heart disease may continue to decline as individuals become more aware of risk factors and accept responsibility for managing their own health.

    c. Diabetes-related mortality is almost 2.5 times higher for Native Americans than for the general population. Black women have higher rates than whites and black men. Diabetes also contributes to coronary artery disease and significantly increases mortality from acute myocardial infarction.

C. Morbidity

1. Hospitalizations

    a. More women than men are hospitalized annually.

    b. In general, the longest hospital stays are for cerebrovascular disease (10.9 days), followed by fractures (9.4 days), malignant neoplasms (8.3 days), and diseases of the heart (7.2 days).

2. Chronic conditions and limitations

    a. Chronic conditions such as arthritis, hypertension, and impairment of the back or spine are more likely to decrease women's activity level than men's.

    b. Almost twice as many women as men are limited in activity level because of arthritis.

3. Surgery

    a. About 25% of all births are by cesarean section, making this the most prevalent surgical procedure experienced by women in the United States.

    b. Hysterectomy is the most frequently performed operation among nonpregnant women ages 15 years and older. Uterine fibroids, endometriosis, uterine prolapse, and cancer are the most common reasons for hysterectomies.

D. Mental health

1. Depression is the most frequent threat to the mental health of women. The symptoms experienced range from feelings of sadness to thoughts of death.

2. Young women (ages 25 to 44) have twice the rate of depression as men of the same age.

E. Other factors

1. Education and work

    a. Nearly 75% of women ages 25 and older are high school graduates (up from 55.4% in 1970).

    b. Seventeen percent of women ages 25 and older have completed college (compared with 8.2% in 1970).

    c. More women are receiving professional degrees than ever before.

2. Employment and wages

    a. Nearly half of the women in the U.S. labor force are working mothers with children less than 6 years of age.

    b. Women earn only $.70 for every $1.00 earned by men.

    c. The poorest aggregate in the United States is women with children. This has been termed the "feminization of poverty."

    d. Nurses working with these families should be aware of social services, child care programs, emergency services, and other resources for families in need.

3. Working women at home

    a. The burden of housework and child care usually falls on women.

    b. These multiple role demands contribute to stress.

    c. This pattern appears to be changing somewhat, however, as younger husbands and fathers assist with a larger portion of family activities and household chores.

4. Family configuration and marital relationship status

    a. Because of diverse family configurations, women's roles within the family are changing.

    b. Many women are delaying marriage or are not marrying.

    c. About 30% of "families" consist of single-parent households, although this varies markedly among ethnic and racial groups. About 63% of African-American families are single-parent families with children at home, compared with 35% of Hispanics and 25% of whites.

5. Health behavior
   a. Women tend to seek information that allow them to be in control of their own health.
   b. Self-help activities include recognizing of signs of STDs, understanding the importance of nutrition, being aware of contraceptive choices, and performing breast self-examination and pregnancy testing.
   c. Knowledge deficits prevail among women regardless of socioeconomic or educational level. Nurses can encourage women to develop a greater sense of self awareness and to play a more active role in their health maintenance.
6. Health care access
   a. About 32 million Americans have no health insurance.
   b. Individuals between the ages of 16 and 24 are disproportionately without any type of health insurance.
   c. For women between the ages of 15 and 44, 28.5% of Hispanics, 21% of blacks, and 15% of whites are without coverage.
   d. Although the elderly are usually covered under Medicare, they often delay seeking health care.

II. Types of Problems
A. Acute illness
   1. Females report a greater incidence of acute conditions than do males.
   2. Diseases of the urinary tract and illnesses specific to the reproductive tract are very common among women.
B. Chronic disease
   1. Cardiovascular disease, hypertension, diabetes, arthritis, osteoporosis, breast conditions, and cancer are chronic diseases that may affect women for many years.
   2. Black women are more vulnerable than white women to arteriosclerotic heart disease (ASHD). Several modifiable risk factors are associated with ASHD, including elevated serum lipid levels; habitual diet high in calories, total fats, cholesterol, and sodium; hypertension; obesity; glucose intolerance; and cigarette smoking.
   3. Hypertension is more common in women than in men and affects more blacks than whites. Hypertension is usually asymptomatic. Therefore, all women should be screened every two years.

4. Screening for diabetes is important for all women. There are approximately 4 million undiagnosed diabetics in the United States.
5. Arthritis is slightly higher in females than in males, but rheumatoid arthritis afflicts three times as many women as men.
6. Osteoporosis is a major disorder that affects postmenopausal women. About 80% of cases are among women. Between 25 and 50% of American women will develop osteoporosis.
7. Breast cancer has increased over the past 50 years, and approximately 1 out of every 9 women will develop breast cancer. Risk factors include age of more than 50, personal or family history of breast cancer, never having had children or having a first child after age 30, obesity, and a diet high in fat. To lower the risk of breast cancer, breast self-examination (BSE) should be taught in high school. Mammography should be done by age 40 for a baseline, every 1 to 2 years for women age 40 to 49, and yearly thereafter.
8. Cancer of the cervix is the most common form of cancer in the genital tract. Risk factors for cervical cancer include coitus before the age of 20, multiple sex partners, history of human papillomavirus, and other STDs. The decline in deaths due to cervical cancer is directly related to early detection through an annual pelvic examination including a pap smear, which should begin when women become sexually active or when they reach age 18.
9. Endometrial cancer has increased during the past 30 years. Eighty percent of women with this condition are postmenopausal. Risk factors include obesity, low parity, diabetes, and high circulating estrogen levels.
10. Ovarian cancer accounts for the majority of deaths in the United States due to pelvic malignancy. Approximately 1 out of 70 American women will have ovarian cancer. Risk factors include increasing age, never having had children, and history of breast or endometrial cancer.
C. Reproductive health
   1. Community health nurses perform a variety of services related to women's reproductive health.
      a. They encourage women to reduce cigarette smoking and use of alcohol and other drugs.

b. They encourage better nutrition.
c. They encourage women to pursue better socioeconomic opportunities by various means, including bettering their education to qualify for higher-paying jobs.

2. Pregnancy may motivate women to develop a better awareness of proper nutrition. The community health nurse can take this opportunity to initiate a referral to WIC when appropriate.

3. The community health nurse has frequent opportunities to provide counseling in the area of family planning. More than half of all pregnancies in the United States are unintended, and approximately 15 to 18% of all couples are unintentionally childless.

4. Benefits of family planning services and counseling include prevention of unwanted pregnancy and reduction in the incidence of abortion.

D. Sexually transmitted diseases and HIV
1. Chlamydia is the most common STD in the United States, but gonorrhea is the most frequently reported. Complications from chlamydia and gonorrhea include tubal occlusion, which contributes to infertility; ectopic pregnancy; and neonatal morbidity and mortality. These diseases may also contribute to the spread of HIV.

2. HIV is rapidly increasing among women and babies born to women in high-risk groups. Women at high risk include intravenous drug users who share needles or syringes, prostitutes, those whose sex partners are infected, and participants in unprotected sex.

E. Unintentional injury (accidents)
1. Older women are at increased risk for accidents such as falls. Associated factors include an unsteady gait, reduced vision, and a hazardous environment.

2. Women of all ages with a history of inadequately explained injuries should be evaluated for possible battering. Women from all socioeconomic levels are affected. Community health nurses need to know how to make assessments, provide support, and make referrals to agencies that deal with domestic violence.

F. Disability
1. Although women have more disabilities resulting from acute conditions than men, they have fewer disabilities from chronic conditions because they tend to report their symptoms earlier and receive necessary treatment.

2. Dysmenorrhea is a frequent disability for many women. It is the single greatest cause of absenteeism from school and work among young women.

III. Major Legislation Affecting Women's Health Services
A. Public Health Service Act (1982)—The Public Health Service Act provides for biomedical and health services research, information dissemination, resource development, technical assistance, and service delivery directed at women's health concerns. Family planning, health promotion, and disease prevention activities are enhanced by this act.

B. Civil Rights Act (1964)
1. The Civil Rights Act was amended in 1978 to prohibit discrimination against pregnant women or conditions involving childbirth or pregnancy.

2. Employee benefit plans that provide disability insurance must include disabilities due to pregnancy and childbirth.

3. Sexual harassment is a violation of the Civil Rights act.

C. Social Security Act
1. The Social Security Act provides retirement and disability benefits to workers and survivors, including those who are divorced.

2. Medicare is also a result of the Social Security Act.

D. Occupational Safety and Health Act
1. The Occupational Safety and Health Act was enacted in 1970 to ensure safe and healthful working conditions.

2. Reproductive risks associated with exposure to occupational health hazards include unfavorable reproductive outcomes such as altered fertility, spontaneous abortion, congenital malformations, intrauterine growth retardation, and fetal deaths. Occupational health nurses should be aware of environmental hazards within the workplace and work to minimize or eliminate them.

E. Family and Medical Leave Act (1993)
1. This act allows an employee to obtain twelve weeks of unpaid leave for family and medical reasons (such as personal illness; illness of a child, spouse or parent; birth; or adoption).

2. This act guarantees the same, or equivalent, job on return, along with continuation of health benefits.

IV. Health and Social Services to Promote Women's Health

A. Approximately 5.7 million women of child-bearing age are assisted by Medicaid.
   1. Many women eligible for Medicaid are at high risk for poor pregnancy outcomes because barriers limit access.
   2. There is a need for public awareness of facilities for maternity care and providers who accept Medicaid.
B. Women consumers are requesting more emphasis in the area of health promotion and disease prevention for women's health care. Nurses throughout the country have established collaborative practices with other health professionals to meet this demand.
C. Many private voluntary organizations spend money, time, and energy attempting to increase health awareness among their members as well as to provide direct services to the public.
   1. One of the most effective voluntary efforts assists abused women by providing shelters and safe houses throughout the United States.
   2. Women's organizations such as Urban League, sororities, Junior League, YWCA, and religious denominations have made women's health a major item on their agenda.

V. Roles of the Community Health Nurse

A. Direct care provider—Direct care is usually given in clinics (family planning, obstetrical/gynecological, STD, etc.) and can be comprehensive.
B. Counselor—The counseling role of the community health nurse occurs in almost every interaction in women's health.

VI. Research in Women's Health

A. In 1990, the NIH created the Office of Research on Women's Health.
   1. The organization established a research agenda for women's health.
   2. Major areas for exploration and research among women include health promotion, barriers to care, health education at various literacy levels, differences among women experiencing menopausal symptoms, dysmenorrhea, contraception, infertility, adolescent sexuality, HIV infection and pregnancy, osteoporosis, and domestic violence.
B. In 1991, the NIH began a prospective study called the Women's Health Initiative.
   1. This study includes women of all races and socioeconomic levels to examine major causes of death, disability and frailty.
   2. Specific conditions addressed include heart disease, stroke, cancer, and osteoporosis.

TEACHING STRATEGIES

1. Have students explore nursing and other health care journals for research studies on women's health issues. Ask each student to bring one study to class to discuss. Are there more women's studies available in nursing literature than in medicine psychology, or public health? Are investigators in the area of women's health generally men or women?
2. Invite a guest speaker from the American Cancer Society or Reach for Recovery. Have the speaker include information on breast cancer statistics and discuss prevention, early diagnosis, and treatment. Discuss BSE and mammography and explore the availability of low-cost mammograms.
3. Invite a nurse from a family planning clinic or women's health clinic to discuss issues related to women's health care. Encourage the speaker to include topics such as access to care, choice of contraception, and changes in the incidence and prevalence of disease in the community.

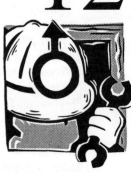

Men's Health

ANNOTATED LEARNING OBJECTIVES

1. Identify the major indicators of men's health status.

The major indicators of men's health status are rates of longevity, mortality, and morbidity. In the United States, men born in 1992 will live an average of 6.8 years less than women. Males in industrialized countries have higher death rates than do females. Men are nearly four times as likely to die from suicide, three times as likely to die from homicide, and twice as likely to die from accidents. Rates of heart disease, some forms of cancer, pneumonia, diabetes, and cerebrovascular diseases are all higher for men than women. Men consistently report better health than women. Women are more likely to be ill (both acute and chronic illnesses), whereas men are more likely to die.

2. Describe two major explanations for men's health status.

Biological factors influence men's health; males have higher rates of infant mortality, congenital anomalies, and chromosome-linked diseases, and they lack the theorized estrogen protection against heart disease enjoyed by women. Biological factors may also contribute to differences in high-risk and aggressive behavior.

Risk-taking behaviors and activities related to socialization (work, leisure, and lifestyle) patterns affect men's health. Men generally have more dangerous occupations, and they have higher rates of traffic fatalities, alcohol consumption, and cigarette smoking, all of which affect health status.

Men's orientation toward illness and prevention affect their health status. Men are less likely than women to seek preventive health care and often fail to limit their activities when they are sick.

3. Discuss factors that impede men's health.

There are very few, if any, practicing health care specialists in men's health. A primary care specialty that focuses specifically on men's needs and sex role influences on health and lifestyle would be beneficial in identifying and avoiding potential and actual threats to health. Access to care, a focus on treatment rather than prevention and promotion, financial considerations, and time limitations all inhibit men from seeking health care.

4. Discuss factors that promote men's health.

Nationally, and in some places internationally, there is a growing interest in men's health issues. Nurses are beginning to define and research matters related to men's health. In recent years, men have become more interested in physical fitness and modifying lifestyle patterns to improve or promote health. There is growing interest in establishing policies and health services specifically directed toward men and men's health issues.

5. Describe men's health needs.

With regard to health, men need permission to have concerns about health and to talk more openly to others about health; consideration of sex role and lifestyle influences on both physical and mental health; information about how their bodies function; self-care instruction; complete history and physical examinations; help with fathering roles; adjustment of the health care system to men's occupational constraints regarding time and location of sources of health care; improvement in financial access to health care; and primary prevention.

6. Apply knowledge of men's health needs in planning sex-appropriate nursing care for males at the individual, family, and community levels.

Nursing care specific for men's health needs should follow the nursing process. Assessment should view the community as a system and focus on systems and subsystems to organize the data. The nurse should perform an individual assessment, as well as an assessment of related issues such as neighborhood, peer groups, work or school environment, church, and civic activities. A nursing diagnosis should be made for each individual, each system component (family), and the aggregate.

Planning involves contracting with aggregates and mutual goal setting. Intervention at the aggregate level calls for group and community work. Examples of interventions with the family include counseling, education, and referral aimed at promoting family self-care. Interventions may also be carried out with other aggregates.

Evaluation is multidimensional and ongoing. Using a systems approach to evaluation, the nurse evaluates each component of the system. Ongoing evaluation includes noting referrals and followup of family and other aggregates in use of resources.

LECTURE OUTLINE

I. **Traditional Indicators of Men's Health Status**
   A. Longevity
      1. Males born in 1992 will live an average of 72.3 years, compared with females who will live an average of 79.1 years.
      2. Life expectancy is associated with socioeconomic status and underserved populations in the United States; minorities, in particular, live significantly fewer years.
         a. Black males will live more than eight years less than white males.
         b. Black females will live almost nine years longer than black males.
      3. A shorter life expectancy for men is common to all contemporary industrialized countries. The United States ranks 25th in life expectancy for men and 16th in life expectancy for women.
   B. Mortality
      1. Males in industrialized countries have higher death rates than do females.
      2. Men are seven times more likely than women to die from AIDS. Men are also four times more likely to die as a result of suicide, three times more likely to die from homicide, and twice as likely to die from accidents, liver disease, or COPD. They are nearly twice as likely to die of pneumonia or diseases of the heart, and they lead in deaths resulting from cancer, kidney disease, cerebrovascular disease, and diabetes.
   C. Morbidity
      1. Men have consistently reported better health than women.
      2. In general, women are more likely to be ill, whereas men are more likely to die.
      3. Acute illness
         a. The incidence rate of acute infective and parasitic disease, respiratory conditions, and digestive conditions is higher for women. The only exception is for injuries, which are around 12% greater for men.
         b. The number of restricted activity days for acute conditions is 33% greater for women than for men, and the number of bed disability days is 38% greater for women than for men.
      4. Chronic conditions
         a. Women are more likely than men to have a higher prevalence of chronic diseases that cause disability and limitation of activities, but do not lead to death.
         b. Men have higher morbidity and mortality rates for conditions that are the leading causes of death.

II. **Use of Medical Care**
   A. Ambulatory care
      1. Men seek ambulatory care less often than do women. Women have approximately 6.2 physician contacts per year, whereas men have 4.3 contacts.
      2. Men are seen more frequently than women for conditions that correspond with their leading mortality causes: ischemic heart disease and cerebrovascular disease.
   B. Hospital care—Discharges from short-stay hospitals were lower for men (9.1 per 100) than for women (12.3 per 100).
   C. Preventive care
      1. Women are more likely than men to receive physical examinations.
      2. Women are more likely to have an ongoing source of care.
   D. Use of other health services
      1. Women are more likely to be admitted for out-patient psychiatric services and to reside

in nursing homes due to their longer life expectancy.
2. Rates of institutionalization in state and county mental hospitals for men is greater than for women.

III. Theories That Explain Men's Health
A. Biological factors
1. Gender differences between men and women are influenced by biological factors including genetics, sex hormones, and physiological differences.
2. Fetal death rates and infant mortality rates due to congenital anomalies are higher for males than for females.
3. Chromosome-linked diseases such as hemophilia, red-green color blindness, and certain types of muscular dystrophy are more common among males.
4. Biological advantages for females may include the protection of estrogen against heart disease.
5. Genetic factors may contribute to gender differences in high-risk and aggressive behavior, mental and penal institutionalization, accidents, and various types of violent deaths.
B. Socialization
1. Risks may be different between males and females due to differences in work, leisure, and lifestyles due to sex roles.
2. Men's occupations tend to be more hazardous and are more likely to include exposure to toxic or carcinogenic substances.
3. Men are at risk for injury from sports and have higher rates of traffic fatalities, alcohol consumption, and cigarette smoking.
C. Orientation toward illness and prevention
1. Women are more likely than men to cut back activities when ill, to seek health care, and to report more details to health care providers.
2. Women are more likely to seek preventive examinations, take vitamins regularly, and brush their teeth.
3. Men are more likely to engage in exercise that is beneficial to cardiovascular health.
D. Reporting health behavior
1. Women are more likely to remember their health problems and actions and to talk with someone about their illness and health.
2. Women recall and report more health problems than do men.
3. Men are typically less willing to talk.
E. Interpreting data

1. All four factors (inherited risks, acquired risks, illness and prevention orientation, and health-reporting behavior) must be considered when interpreting data. The social factors of gender differences in illness and prevention orientations and health-reporting behavior are critical in interpreting health interview data.
2. Conditions that affect morbidity (arthritis and gout) do not significantly affect mortality, and conditions that affect mortality (heart disease) may not cause morbidity.
3. Men and women respond to their health problems differently.
   a. Males have higher prevalence and death rates for disease and injury and accident mortality.
   b. Females have higher prevalence rates for a greater number of nonfatal chronic conditions.
   c. Females tend to take care of themselves when ill, seek preventive help, and talk about health. These factors boost the morbidity rate.
4. The largest gender-related difference in mortality occurs for deaths associated with sex-linked behavior. Sex-linked behaviors that correlate with major causes of death include smoking (lung cancer, emphysema, asthma); alcohol consumption (cirrhosis, accidents, homicide); stress and poor preventive health habits (heart disease); and lack of other emotional channels (suicide, homicide, accidents).

IV. Factors That Impede Men's Health
A. Medical care patterns
1. There are currently no specialists in men's health. In recent years, however, there has been a noticeable effort to reestablish general health care through "family practice" and primary care.
2. Without a primary care specialty that focuses specifically on men's needs, many needs and sex role influences on health and lifestyle may not be addressed by anyone.
B. Access to care
1. Mission orientation
   a. Mission-oriented health care is offered by the military, sports, and some industries to maintain an effective work force.
   b. Overall, however, mission-oriented health care demonstrates a lack of focus on prevention and health promotion at the individual and aggregate levels.

2. Financial considerations
   a. Many insurance companies reimburse only for a diagnosed condition—for pathology, not for preventive care.
   b. Managed care arrangements, which encourage primary care, may improve access for many men.
3. Time factors
   a. Men and women appear to have approximately equal access to health care based on office schedules and provider availability.
   b. Men may be reluctant to take time from work for a medical visit due to loss of income or fear of being seen as weak or ill.
C. Lack of health promotion
   1. The disease focus of the present health care system is limited in addressing the precursors of today's mortalities.
   2. Medical measures have not made substantial impact on mortality due to coronary heart disease, cancer, and stroke (conditions that account for two thirds of all mortality).
   3. An increase in life expectancy has occurred, but has resulted in an increase in years of disability.
   4. The effects of pharmacology, coronary care units, and coronary bypass surgery have been negligible in the reduction of deaths due to coronary heart disease. Rather, changes in lifestyle habits appear to be responsible for the decrease in heart disease deaths.
   5. Similarly, resources for cancer are directed toward cure and treatments rather than prevention.

V. **Factors That Promote Men's Health**
   A. Interest groups in men's health
      1. There is a small, but growing, number of individuals interested in men's health issues.
      2. Nurses are beginning to define and study men's health issues.
   B. Increasing interest in physical fitness and lifestyle
      1. Men's interest in altering behavior that places them at risk of cardiovascular and other major diseases is increasing. Smoking decreased from 51% to 27% of all men between 1965 and 1993.
      2. Men report exercising much more frequently than women.
   C. Policy related to men's health—Nurses are working to set policy related to men's health,

particularly in the area of family planning and fatherhood.
   D. Health services for men
      1. There is a lack of health care clinics that are tailored to the special needs of men.
      2. The development of men's health care facilities may be strongly encouraged by some, but their efforts may fail during the era of managed care.

VI. **Men's Health Care Needs**—Biological and psychosocial causes of men's health show that the following improvements are needed in men's health care.
   A. Permission to have concerns about health and to talk more openly to others about health
   B. Consideration of sex-role and lifestyle influences on their physical and mental health
   C. Information about how their bodies function (what is normal and abnormal, what action to take, proper nutrition, exercise patterns)
   D. Self-care instruction, physical examination, and history-taking that includes sexual and reproductive health
   E. Help with fathering
   F. Adjustment of the health care system to men's occupational constraints regarding time and location of source of health care
   G. Increasing affordability of health care
   H. Primary prevention

VII. **Meeting Men's Health Needs**—Interdisciplinary efforts are needed to address the many factors that affect the health of men.
   A. Traditional health services
      1. Services currently available are diagnostic and treatment-oriented, rather than preventive.
      2. Payment for health services may be out-of-pocket or through private insurance or HMOs.
      3. Health services such as programs that address heart disease, kidney disease, cancer, stroke, and mental health are offered by local and state health departments.
   B. New concepts of community care
      1. Public health care practices that focus on modification of behavioral and lifestyle characteristics that influence health to promote positive influences, and reduce negative ones, are being employed at some locations.
      2. Directing family planning services toward teenage boys and young men has proved successful.

VIII. Application of the Nursing Process
  A. The community health nurse may promote self-care in male members of the family, facilitate men's health by addressing changes at the family level, and bring about changes in policy that affects men at the community level.
  B. Gender-appropriate care for males can be enhanced by the following.
     1. Applying the nursing process at all levels of prevention for individuals, families, and aggregates
     2. Undertaking appropriate roles of the community health nurse in care planning and provision
     3. Participating in research on men's health issues.
  C. Applying the nursing process
     1. Assessment
        a. Assessment should view the community as a system and focus on systems and subsystems to organize the data.
        b. An individual assessment and an assessment of the neighborhood and peer groups, work or school environment, and church and civic activities should be performed.
     2. Diagnosis—A nursing diagnosis is made for each individual, each system component (family), and the aggregate.
     3. Planning
        a. Planning involves contracting with aggregates and mutual goal-setting.
        b. Planning is an outcome of mutually derived assessment and diagnosis.
        c. Mutual goal setting requires collaboration on long- and short-term goals.
     4. Intervention
        a. Intervention at the aggregate level calls for group and community work.
        b. Examples of interventions with the family include counseling, education, and referral aimed at promoting family self-care.
        c. Interventions must also be carried out with other aggregates.
     5. Evaluation
        a. Evaluation is multidimensional and ongoing.
        b. Using a systems approach to evaluation, the nurse evaluates each component of the system.
        c. Ongoing evaluation includes noting referrals and followup of family and other aggregates in use of resources.

IX. Roles of the Community Health Nurse
  A. Health educator
     1. Health educational efforts should focus on tailoring messages to the needs of men.
     2. Education can address the need to change societal attitudes that encourage negative health behaviors, including risk-taking among males.
  B. Facilitator
     1. Facilitating change by promoting healthy life-long behaviors by parents and other family members is important.
     2. The community health nurse may also facilitate change at the aggregate level by assessing the community's needs and resources specifically designed for men.
     3. The community health nurse needs to join organizations and create awareness of men's health as an issue.
     4. A review of nursing and other professional literature for issues related to men's health and a review of indexes in nursing texts for men's health or men's reproductive health and/or fathering may be helpful.

X. Research and Men's Health—Community health nurses must work to ensure a safe workplace and environment for both men and women. Community health nurses also provide for the disadvantaged who may not have the economic freedom to choose from a range of options. Research directed toward men's health might answer some concerns. Health aspects of men's roles in the family, in childbearing, and in parenting are needed. A cross-disciplinary approach would be helpful to include social and psychological dimensions.

XI. Web Resources on Men's Health
  A. The Diagnostic Center for Men
     1. (http://www.for-men.com/comit.htm/)
     2. A national network of diagnostic clinics that evaluate and treat men for sexual dysfunction
  B. WWW Virtual Library—Men's Health
     1. (http://info-sys.home.vix.com/men/health/health.htm/)
     2. Articles, bibliographies, and links to other web sites regarding physical and mental health and legislation
  C. Circumcision Facts
     1. (http://www.gepps.com/circ.htm/)
     2. Pros and cons, links to other resources and support organizations
  D. Impotence Resource Center
     1. (http://www.impotence.org/)

2. Information, bookstore, newsletter
E. Stop AIDS Project
1. (http://www.stopaids.org/)
2. Resources for gay and bisexual men
F. Prostatitis Home Page
1. (http://www.prostate.org/)
2. Information and fact sheets from the Prostatitis Foundation
G. Men's Health Daily
1. (http://www.menshealth.com/)
2. Online companion to the printed magazine *Men's Health,* which is sold at newsstands

TEACHING STRATEGIES

1. Have students review nursing research journals to identify recent studies dealing specifically with research of men's health issues. Have them bring photocopies to class to discuss. What issues are being addressed? What issues are not being addressed? What areas need to be stressed for further research?

2. Have male students lead a discussion on men's health and what is missing in the current health care system. What can nurses do to improve health care delivery for this aggregate?

Addressing the Needs of Families

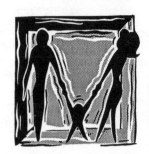

ANNOTATED LEARNING OBJECTIVES

1. State a personal definition of "family."

The word *family* can be defined structurally, such as a cluster of people who live together in a relationship of marriage and descent; culturally, which may include the extended family both laterally (grandparents, aunt, uncles, cousins) and vertically (descendants and ancestors); or functionally, where family members meet individual needs through the performance of various roles.

In the United States, the "typical" family is the nuclear family, which is a small group consisting of parents and their non-adult children living in a single household. However, this view of the family accounts for less than half of the households in the United States.

2. Identify characteristics of the changing family that have implications for community health nursing practice.

The increasing number of single-parent families, in particular those headed by single mothers, is very important in planning community health nursing care. Families headed by single women are much more likely to be in poverty and are disproportionately represented by minorities. The limited income of single-parent families has implications for health, particularly in relation to access to health care and use of preventive services. The poor nutrition, substandard housing, and general living conditions seen in poverty also tend to be detrimental to health.

3. Describe strategies for moving from intervention at the individual level to intervention at the family level.

There are many tools and strategies to assist the community health nurse in providing family-level interventions. Family interviewing is a tool for caring for the family as a whole. In family interviewing the nurse cares for the family through use of general systems theory and family assessment to assess the family's response to events such as births, retirement, chronic illness, or divorce.

Nurses working in clinics can assess the health of the individual as a part of the family. School nurses can compare a child in the school system with the child in the family system. Assessment of needs of children as a part of their families or as an individual at school can lead to interventions such as support groups for learning or behavior problems, absenteeism, or care for chronic illness.

Occupational health nurses can assess occupational hazards including reproductive problems, stress, and injuries. Screening, referral, and health education of the employee and family members can contribute to the overall health and well being for the employee and can therefore be beneficial to the employer.

Intervention during chronic illness can address changes in family patterns, fears, and emotional responses. Special needs of the primary caretaker, such stress or fatigue, can be addressed to influence family interaction positively.

4. Describe strategies for moving from intervention at the family level to intervention at the aggregate level.

The community health nurse should view families as components of communities, and the nurse must know the community. The community should be assessed and analyzed in terms of differences in health needs, differences in resources, and ways to impact health policy and redistribute resources to meet health needs. Through the community assessment process, the nurse can compare census tracts with city, county, state, and national data on health statistics. As differences between major health needs from one subpopulation differ greatly from others, cross-comparison of the communities and the needs of the families are necessary. These can then be used to set priorities for delivery of health care.

5. *Discuss the application of one conceptual framework to studying families.*

General systems theory can be used to explain how the family as a unit interacts with larger units outside the family and with smaller units inside the family. The family may be affected by any disrupting force acting on the system outside it or on a system within it (subsystem). The family is seen as a system in balance, but one that may become unbalanced at any time. Systems concepts can be used to explain family functioning and provide direction for intervention.

A structural-functional conceptual framework views the family according to the structure of the parts of its system. Internal structure of the family is the family composition, order, subgroups, or dyads through which the family functions. External structure is the larger context of the family, including the culture, religion, social class, environment, home, and extended family. Functional structure refers to how family members behave toward each other. Interventions can be directed to either the structural or functional areas as needed.

6. *Discuss a model of care for communities of families.*

A number of models guide provision of care that is accessible, equal, and sensitive to all individuals, families, and aggregates. Care should be comprehensive and accessible, encourage family participation, and use a team approach. Alternative programs can change the structural barriers that prevent access to care for low-income families. Professional role functions may be altered as nurses, rather than physicians, provide health care. Active self-care should be promoted, and health and medical knowledge should be shared. Assistance by family and social networks is encouraged. Social changes may be necessary to improve the health of the underserved populations.

7. *Apply the steps of the nursing process to individuals within the family, to the family as a whole, and to an aggregate of which the family is a part.*

Assessment—The nurse should assess and reassess the family in their home environment and within the neighborhood. A systems theory approach can be helpful in organizing the data collection. The nurse should assess verbal and nonverbal cues, as well as environmental and behavioral information; observe family dynamics, including communication patterns among family members, roles taken, and the division of labor. Assessment should also include the resources available to the family in terms of social support, schools, recreation, and religious activities.

Diagnosis—Nursing diagnosis can be made for each individual family member and for the family as a whole. Nursing diagnoses may stem from a structural/functional framework, systems framework, problems in communication, or roles and value conflicts.

Planning—Planning with the family is essential and involves mutual goal setting between nurse and family; mutual setting of objectives to meet goals; prioritizing; and contracting to establish the division of labor between the nurse and the family.

Intervention—Interventions offered by the nurse are those directed to the family functioning at the cognitive, affective, and behavioral levels.

Evaluation—Evaluation is the ongoing process of observing family progress toward meeting goals identified by the nurse and family.

LECTURE OUTLINE

The individual is the unit most frequently addressed by all components of the health care system, including nursing. However, nurses are working toward enhancing interventions directed at the family level.

I. **The Changing Family**
   A. Definition of the family
      1. The term *family* is defined as
         a. "A social unit interacting with the larger society"
         b. "A cluster of people whose relationship is stipulated by law in terms of marriage and descent, and whose precise membership varies according to the circumstances"
         c. "A primary group of people living in a household in consistent proximity and intimate relationship"
      2. In addition, the family may be defined culturally.
         a. White Americans tend to define family in terms of the intact nuclear family.
         b. African-Americans focus on the extended family.
         c. Chinese include ancestors and all their descendants.

d. Italians may include several generations including godparents and old friends.

B. Characteristics of the changing family

1. The "typical" family—the nuclear family—is defined as "a small group consisting of parents and their non-adult children living in a single household."

2. This stereotypical view of the family is eroding, however, with only 70% of today's children living with two parents (1994). This is particularly striking among black children, among whom only 36% live with two parents.

3. Cohabitation has increased more than 500% in the past 30 years.

4. Single-parent families, particularly mother-only households, have increased greatly in the past two decades.

   a. The effect of single-parent families on income is dramatic; mother-only households have approximately one-third the income of households with two parents.

   b. Over half of mother-only black families and one-third of mother-only white families live below the poverty level.

II. **Approaches to Meeting the Health Needs of Families**

A. Nursing in a family context

1. Community health nurses should be aware that the individual can best be understood within the social context of the family.

2. Direct intervention at the family level, rather than the individual client level, is new to most nurses.

3. Birthing, parent-child relationships, adult day care, chronic illness, and home care are best addressed using nursing practice models emphasizing the family.

B. Moving from the individual to the family

1. Reimbursement is calculated for services rendered to the individual and is a major constraint in moving toward planning care for families. Therefore, the community health nurse needs a variety of creative approaches to meeting the health needs of families.

2. Family interviewing

   a. Care of families should be creative, flexible and transferable from one setting to another. Family interviewing is a model for caring for the family as a whole.

   b. The community health nurse uses general systems and communication concepts

to conceptualize the health needs of families and a family assessment model to assess families' responses to events such as births, retirement, chronic illness, or divorce.

   c. Family interviewing requires thinking in terms of the family system and in terms of the larger social system.

   d. Clinical settings appropriate for family interviewing include inpatient and outpatient ambulatory care and clinic settings in maternity, pediatrics, medicine, surgery, critical care, and mental health.

   e. Community health nurses have many opportunities to engage families in interviews. In each case, community health nurses can assess and intervene at the family and community levels.

   f. The school nurse has a unique opportunity to compare the child in the school system with the child in the family system. Assessment of needs of children within the context of their families in an interview at school or in the home can lead to innovative interventions such as support groups for children with chronic illness and interventions in areas such as learning or behavior problems and absenteeism.

   g. The occupational health nurse can use a family approach to improve the health of the worker and contribute to overall productivity. Assessment of occupational hazards may involve conducting reproductive histories in an effort to determine the effects of a chemical or agent on the reproductive capacity of the couple. Obtaining an occupational history from all family members who have entered the workplace, referral for screening, and health education of family members will contribute to identifying and reducing occupational hazards.

   h. In cases of chronic illness, interventions by the community health nurse are aided by the family interview. Changes in family patterns, fears, emotional responses, and expectations of individual family members can be assessed.

C. Moving from the family to the community

1. In addition to providing care to individuals and families, the community health nurse should provide care to communities.

2. Families must be viewed as components of communities, and the nurse must know the community.

3. The community must be assessed and analyzed in terms of differences in health needs, differences in resources to effect interventions, and ways to impact policy and redistribute resources to ensure that the health needs of the families and communities are met.

4. Physical, social, and demographic data provide an empirical basis for the development and delivery of nursing services. Community health nurses can compare city data with county, state, and national data. They should be aware that specific health needs vary among census tracts. The major health needs of one subpopulation will differ from those of others.

5. In addition to the cross-comparison of communities, the community health nurse must also cross-compare the needs of families within the communities. Just as specific health needs vary among census tracts, so too do health needs vary among families.

III. **The Family Theory Approach to Meeting the Health Needs of Families**

A. Reasons for working with families

1. A dysfunction within the family that affects one or more family members will affect other family members and the family as a whole.

2. The wellness of the family is dependent on the role of the family

3. The level of wellness of the family can be raised through care that reduces lifestyle and environmental risks by emphasizing health promotion, self-care, health education, and family counseling

4. Commonalities in risk factors can lead to case finding within the family; and a clear understanding of the functioning of the individual can be gained only when the individual is assessed within the larger context of the family.

B. Systems approach

1. General systems theory is a way to explain how the family as a unit interacts with larger units outside the family and with smaller units inside the family.

   a. A family may be affected by any disrupting force that acts on a system outside of it (suprasystem) or on a system within it (subsystem).

   b. The family is seen as a system hopefully in balance, but which may become unbalanced at any time.

   c. Stabilizing forces from other parts of the system may reestablish balance.

2. Systems concepts can be combined with communication theory to explain family functioning and provide direction for intervention.

3. Certain family member characteristics contribute to healthy families as systems.

   a. Members who interact with each other repeatedly in many contexts

   b. Members who are enhanced and fulfilled by maintaining contact with a wide range of community groups and organizations

   c. Members who make efforts to master their lives by becoming members of other groups

   d. Members who engage in flexible role relationships, share power, respond to change, and support the growth and autonomy of others

C. Structural-functional conceptual framework— In this framework, a family is viewed according to its structure (the parts of the system) and according to its function (what the family does and in what context).

1. Structural

   a. *Internal structure* of the family refers to family composition, rank order, and subsystem, or labeling the subgroups or dyads through which the family carries out its functions and boundary.

   b. *External structure* refers to the larger context of the family and includes the culture, religion, social class status and mobility, environment or neighborhood, and home and extended family.

   c. *Context* refers to background or situation relevant to an event in which the family system is nested and includes ethnicity, race, social class, religion, and environment.

2. Functional

   a. *Functional structure* refers to how family members behave toward each other.

   b. *Instrumental function* describes activities of daily living.

   c. *Expressive function* includes emotional components. Communication patterns, problem solving abilities, roles, control, and alliances and coalition within the family are examples of expressive functions.

3. Developmental
   a. A normal family experiences several developmental stages.
   b. The "typical" family goes through the developmental stages of launching, marriage, families with young children, families with adolescents, families as launching centers, and aging families.

4. Alterations in family development: divorce and remarriage
   a. Alterations to life-cycle occur with separation, divorce, single parenting, and remarriage.
   b. In divorce, post-divorce, and remarriage the family must engage in emotional work.

D. Tools to assist the community health nurse in assessing the family
   1. A *genogram* can help the nurse outline the family's structure by diagramming the family constellation. The genogram may be used during an early family interview and includes births, deaths, divorces, and remarriages.
   2. A *family health tree* is another tool that may be used by the community health nurse. By expanding on the genogram, the family health tree provides a way to record the family's medical and health histories.
      a. Causes of death of deceased family members, when known, are important.
      b. Genetically linked diseases, including heart disease, cancer, diabetes, hypertension, sickle cell anemia, allergies, asthma, and mental retardation are particularly important to assess.
      c. Environmental and occupational diseases, psychosocial problems such as mental illness and obesity, and infectious disease should be noted.
      d. From health problems, the nurse can note familial risk factors.
      e. The family health tree can be used to plan or enhance positive familial influences on risk factors such as diet, exercise, coping with stress, or pressure to have a physical examination.
   3. An *ecomap* is a tool that is used to depict a family's linkages to its suprasystems.
      a. The ecomap shows the connections between the family and the world.

   b. The ecomap points to conflicts to be mediated and resources to be sought.
   c. The ecomap should be completed during an early family interview and should note people, institutions, and agencies significant to the family.

4. A *family health assessment* helps identify the health status of individual members of the family and aspects of family composition, function, and process. A family health assessment may elicit information about the environment or community context, as well as the family, and enables the community health nurse to plan interventions appropriately.

5. *Social and structural constraints* may prevent families from receiving care. It is therefore important to assess for these constraints when planning for family interventions.
   a. Constraints are usually based on social and economic factors that affect a wide range of conditions associated with major health indicators (mortality and morbidity). Literacy, education, and employment are examples.
   b. Constraints common to the health care system include hours of service, distance and transportation, availability of interpreters, and criteria for receiving services (i.e., age, gender, and income barriers).
   c. Helping families understand constraints and linking them to accessible resources are vital activities.

IV. **Extending Family Health Intervention to Larger Aggregates and Social Action**
A. Institutional context of family therapists—Most family theories view the family as a system that interacts with outside suprasystems or institutions only when there is a problem to be addressed. The interaction between the family and the larger social system is addressed by some approaches.
   1. The *ecological approach* focuses on a complex and flexible structure that helps families overcome rigid boundaries and initiate procedures that help them maintain themselves in their environment.
   2. *Network therapy* involves changing the network (extended family or friends) who tend to maintain dysfunction in the nuclear family. This is done by replacing the dysfunctional network with another from the suprasystem that provides more support and

therefore enhances the functioning of the family.

3. The *transactional field* approach sees the family as an institution culturally set in other institutions, such as religious, educational, recreational, and governmental settings.

   a. An awareness of the culture of each system and exploration of the value patterns of the family is important.

   b. An awareness of the culture of origin, changing family values, and the family's interpretation of U.S. values is essential to viewing the interaction of systems with each other.

B. Models of social class and health services

1. There is evidence that social class and race place major limitations on access to medical care.

2. Approximately 20% of the U.S. population is uninsured or underinsured.

3. Children, those with family incomes less than $14,000, those residing in the south, and ethnic/racial minorities are most often without health care coverage.

4. Culture of poverty explains that the relationship between social class and health service is due to a crisis orientation, living-for-the-moment attitude, health beliefs that are culturally transmitted, a low value of health, and an external locus of control.

5. The structural view of use of health care services considers two sets of constraints that limit use of health care.

   a. Lack of financial resources

   b. Characteristics of health care settings for the poor

6. Unequal health care is more a result of the system of care rather than of individual characteristics of people seeking care.

7. Systems barriers tend to be more of a deterrent than inadequate financial coverage.

C. Models of care for communities of families

1. Some models guide provision of care that is accessible and equal and sensitive.

2. Care should have the following characteristics.

   a. Be comprehensive

   b. Encourage family participation

   c. Be accessible

   d. Use a team approach

3. Alternative programs should change the structural barriers that prevent access to care for low-income families.

4. Professional roles may change as nurses, rather than physicians, provide health care.

5. Promoting active self-care and sharing of health and medical knowledge are components of the care of families.

6. Assistance by family and social networks should be encouraged.

V. **Application of the Nursing Process**

A. The home visit

1. Characteristics of home health care

   a. Providing health care in the home to people who have an identified health problem has been shown to be less expensive than hospital care.

   b. Due to limited public health resources, home visiting to well families is largely limited to high-risk populations such as primiparous mothers and their infants and infants at risk for developmental disabilities.

   c. Setting priorities and visiting families in the community is necessary.

   d. A home visit is usually initiated by a referral from a clinic, a school, a private physician, or an agency responsible for care of a particular aggregate.

2. The nursing process in home health care

   a. Assessment

      1) The nurse should assess and reassess the family in its home environment and within the neighborhood.

      2) A systems theory approach, in which the community is the suprasystem and the family is a system composed of subsystems, can help organize data collection.

      3) Data about the family should be collected from as many members of the family as possible.

      4) The nurse should assess verbal and nonverbal cues, as well as environmental and behavioral information.

      5) The nurse should observe family dynamics, including communication patterns among family members, roles taken, and division of labor.

      6) Assessment should include resources such as social support, schools, recreation, and religious activities available to the family.

   b. Diagnosis

      1) Nursing diagnoses can be made for each individual family member and for the family as a whole.

2) Nursing diagnoses may stem from a structural/functional framework, a systems framework, problems in communication, or roles and value conflicts.

c. Planning—Planning with the family is essential. It involves the nurse and family working together to set mutual goals, to set objectives to meet those goals; and prioritizing and contracting to establish the division of labor between the nurse and the family.

d. Intervention—Interventions are directed to family function at the cognitive, affective, and behavioral levels.

1) Cognitive intervention provides new information to the family to promote problem solving.

2) Affective intervention encourages families to express emotions that may block their efforts at problem solving.

3) Behavioral intervention tasks are assigned to be carried out during the family interview.

e. Evaluation—Evaluation is the ongoing process of observing family progress toward meeting goals identified by the nurse and family.

TEACHING STRATEGIES

1. Have students compose a definition of family. Divide the class into groups of five or six students and discuss criteria for a family. Are the criteria based on culture, structure, or function? Have each group share its findings with the larger group.

2. Have each student complete a genogram, family health tree, and/or ecomap on his or her own family. Ask students to identify potential areas for intervention at the individual and family levels. Have them share with the rest of the class on a voluntary basis.

3. Ask each student to identify a family from their clinical experiences who are at risk for dysfunction. If the family is agreeable, have the students complete a family health assessment on the family and make nursing diagnoses and recommendations. Have several students share their findings with the class.

Senior Health

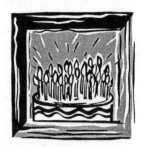

ANNOTATED LEARNING OBJECTIVES

1. *Identify the major indicators of senior health.*

Major indicators of health of the elderly are mortality, morbidity, health behavior and health care, income, literacy and education, marital status, relationships and living arrangements, and religion.

2. *Describe the problems associated with aging.*

Most problems associated with aging arise from the deterioration of physical and/or mental abilities. Problems include difficulties at home (i.e., difficulty in meeting nutritional needs, housework, shopping); disability (which influences an elder's ability to care for him/herself); accidents; use and misuse of medications; and susceptibility to problems imposed by thermal stress.

Problems posed by illness and hospitalization include the fact that hospitalization is a major disruption of everyday life for the elder. Because of DRGs, hospitals discharge patients very quickly, and they are sent home ill. Institutionalization is usually the last resort when the family is no longer able to care for an individual.

Death and bereavement are a part of aging in which people loose their parents, spouses, siblings, friends, and possibly children. The community environment may present problems for the aged. Transportation, safety factors, availability of shopping facilities, and health care are of concern. Abuse of the elderly by caregivers is becoming more common, and the elderly are easy targets for crime.

3. *Discuss the factors that promote senior health.*

Prevention of health problems is the best way to promote senior health. Promotion of senior health includes provision of adequate nutrition; limiting disability through use of health care providers and services; interventions to prevent accidents by assessing the home environment to eliminate hazards; outlining a plan for taking medications to reduce overdosing and underdosing; and ensuring that the elderly have adequate heat in the winter and ways to stay cool in the summer. In addition, screening and case-finding are important to prevent, identify, or control chronic disease. Preventive measures such as immunizations can be used to reduce death and illness from influenza and pneumonia.

4. *Coordinate support services for the elderly.*

Many services are available for the elderly through the Administration on Aging, the Social Security Administration, the Health Care Financing Administration, and local senior citizens centers. The community health nurse working with elderly clients should be aware of resources available in the area; how to refer clients to those resources; requirements for eligibility; and source of payment. Knowledge of local services such as home-delivered meals, assistance with utility bills, and transportation are necessary for nurses working with this aggregate.

5. *Plan appropriate nursing care for seniors in the community.*

When applying the nursing process to seniors, care should be taken to ensure that data collection is complete and systematic. Nutrition, elimination, activity, medication consumption, body protection, cognitive tasks, life changes, the environment, the family, and the community of the client should all be assessed. Diagnoses are based on the individual client's needs and problems. Sharing and validation of diagnoses with clients and mutual setting of goals and objectives will assist in compliance. Planning should be theory-based and directed by mutual goals and objectives. The nurse should work with the client, the family, other care providers, and the community when implementing the plan. Evaluation should be ongoing and jointly accomplished by the nurse, client, and family. It should be used as a tool to direct further interventions.

6. ***Discuss allocation of resources for senior health.***
    Allocation of limited health care resources is an extremely important ethical consideration, particularly when applied to health care provision for the elderly. Effective and equitable distribution of health care resources is very difficult when funds are limited. Should more funds be directed toward caring for the young and less toward treatment of the elderly, where limited benefit of treatment can be seen? In the next several decades, as the elderly become a much higher percentage of the population, more financial resources will be needed to meet health care and other needs. Biomedical ethics and public policy must address the dilemma of who receives health care, for how long, and when care should be removed.

LECTURE OUTLINE

The first goal of Healthy People 2000 *is to increase the span of healthy life. The goal of health care for the elderly is to maximize the ability to perform activities of daily living (ADLs) rather than to focus on cure of pathology. Health care for elders requires a team approach that includes professionals from many different disciplines, and the nurse may be the most important member of the team by providing the leadership necessary for a care-based orientation.*

I. Major Indicators of Health in the Elderly
  A. Aging is defined by chronological age.
     1. The elderly are considered to be people age 65 or older, with people between the ages of 65 and 74 being the "young old," those ages 75-84 being the "older-elderly," and those age 85 or older the "older ages" or "oldest old."
     2. The "frail elderly" are elderly people who are dependent on others for day-to-day care.
  B. Elderly population in the United States
     1. The aggregate of the elderly is the most rapidly expanding section of the U.S. population, growing from 4% in 1900 to 12.5% in 1990 and projected to be 20.4% by 2050. By 2050, it is estimated that 5% of the total population will be composed of those age 85+.
     2. The states with the largest elderly populations are California, Florida, New York, Penn-

sylvania, Texas, Illinois, Ohio, Michigan, and New Jersey.
     3. Approximately 86% of the elderly are non-Hispanic whites, and 13.5% are minorities.
     4. The implications of this growth present an enormous challenge to future government policy-makers because the elderly are the greatest users of health services and various systems of support.
  C. Mortality
     1. In the United States, life expectancy is about 75.7 years and varies by gender and race, with the mortality rate for men exceeding women at every stage of life.
     2. The leading cause of death for people aged 65+ is heart disease. Cancer is the second leading cause of death for those 65+, and cerebrovascular disease and stroke are the third leading cause of death.
     3. The major acute causes of death are influenza, pneumonia, and accidents.
  D. Morbidity
     1. Morbidity statistics indicate quality of life. These statistics can direct the nurse's focus in planning for better health for the aggregate.
     2. Many of the elderly suffer from one or more chronic and degenerative diseases.
        a. Arthritis affects almost half the elderly population.
        b. Hypertension, hearing impairment, heart conditions, cataracts, diabetes, urinary tract diseases, hemorrhoids, and constipation are common conditions in the elderly.
        c. Many elderly people are hospitalized for acute episodes of chronic conditions, with hospitalization being most common for neoplasm and cardiac, circulatory system, digestive, and respiratory diseases.
     3. There are two views on long-term morbidity and aging.
        a. One view indicates that improved health in younger years will continue into old age and compress the degeneration associated with aging into a short period before death.
        b. Another view is that people will merely live longer with chronic disease, which will require increased funding for health care services as the population ages.
  E. Health behavior and health care
     1. Continued good health is the major concern of the elderly.

a. Health is considered good if lifestyle is not affected by physical or mental incapacity.
b. People 65+ are less likely than younger persons to smoke, be overweight, use alcohol to excess, and state that stress has contributed to poor health.
c. Poor health threatens independence and loss of control over lifestyle and warns of imminent death.
d. The most necessary requirements for continued health are a nutritious diet and sufficient exercise to maintain good heart function and increase bone strength.
2. Social and psychological fitness are manifested by relationships, friends, and continued goals for life.
3. Dental needs of elders are often neglected, usually for financial reasons.
a. About half of the elderly have no natural teeth.
b. The loss of teeth leads to poor nutrition and causes a change in body image, loss of self-esteem, and withdrawal from social networks.
4. Aging does not necessarily result in a decline in mental health, but the elderly with mental health problems are often neglected.
a. Mental health problems are one of the principal reasons for institutionalization as people grow older.
b. Suicide is a more frequent cause of death in the elderly than in any other age group.
c. Depression is observed in up to 15% of elders.
d. Community mental health resources for the elderly are lacking.
F. Income
1. Social Security benefits are the major source of income for the elderly, providing more than half of the total income for the majority of recipients. About 25% of recipients derive almost all of their income from this source.
2. Earnings interest on savings and pension plans from other organizations provide other income.
3. Poverty is most likely to occur in households headed by women and minorities.
G. Literacy and education
1. The elderly have less formal schooling than later generations.
a. In 1989, the median education received by the elderly was 12 years.
b. About half of the elderly have completed high school.
2. Whites have a higher educational level than nonwhites.
3. About 2% of the elderly are unable to read and write, and probably more than 20–25% are functionally illiterate.
H. Marital status and living arrangements
1. Because women live longer than men, most older men are married (74%) and most older women are widowed (49%).
2. Most elderly men live in a family, whereas most elderly women live alone.
3. Most of the elderly (about 70%) have surviving children and report living fairly close to at least one.
4. Increasing numbers of the very old are dependent on children who are also elderly. As a result, young family members may find themselves caring for two older generations.
5. Most elderly people own their own homes; about 25% rent, and only about 5% of the elderly live in institutions such as nursing homes.
I. Religion
1. The elderly are more likely than most age groups to participate in church activities. Church membership is claimed by 73% of women and 63% of men 50+.
2. Religious institutions have responded to the needs of older people in their congregations by providing many services to assist them.
3. The parish nurse role is one trend that is expanding steadily.
II. **Problems of the Elderly**—Most problems with aging arise from deterioration of physical and/or mental abilities possessed in the younger years. Health in the elderly has been described as the ability to live and function effectively in society and to exercise self-determination.
A. Difficulties at home
1. Nutrition
a. Consistent, good nutrition is probably the greatest single contribution to physical and mental health and gives the greatest return for the money and time invested.
b. Nutrition needs of the elderly are difficult to assess.
c. Recommended dietary allowances have not been made for the elderly.

d. If food is not appealing and there is no desire to eat, nutrition is not likely to be adequate.

e. Loneliness, depression, grief, and anxiety are common reasons for altered eating habits.

f. It is a challenge for nurses to identify the nutritional adequacy of food consumed by elderly clients.

2. Disability

a. Disability turns routine activities of daily living into time-consuming challenges and is a source of constant irritation for elderly people if mobility and communication with the outside world are affected.

b. Examples of disability include difficulty breathing (caused by emphysema), deficiencies caused by stroke, deformities of arthritis and osteoporosis, incontinence, and loss of vision and/or hearing.

3. Accidents

a. Accidents that cause injury and injury-related deaths are fairly common in the elderly.

b. Reduced sensory perception, increased reaction time, circulatory changes resulting in dizziness or loss of balance, and confusion make the elderly "accident prone."

c. Primary prevention includes assessment of the environment and intervention to avoid accidents.

d. Eliminating environmental hazards, reducing the hot water heater setting, checking the kitchen stove, and ensuring that fire extinguishers are accessible and that smoke detectors function correctly can help prevent accidents and injuries.

4. Medications

a. Both prescription and nonprescription medications are commonly used by the elderly.

b. The effects of different drugs on the aging population is unknown in many cases, and drug dosage is achieved through trial and error.

c. Little attention is given to possible drug-drug or drug-food interaction.

d. Even if the most appropriate medications are prescribed, they are often not used as directed.

e. Medications may be discontinued when symptoms disappear, they may be over-consumed, they may be forgotten, or they may have never been purchased if money is scarce.

f. Ten times as many deaths from accidental poisoning may occur in the elderly than in children. This may be partially due to combined effects of drugs and alcohol or from an unintentional drug overdose following confusion or forgetfulness.

g. Medications should not be kept by the bedside, outdated medications should be discarded, and a plan should be devised to assist the client in taking medications only as prescribed.

5. Thermal stress

a. Thermal stress caused by heat exhaustion or hypothermia is due to the elder's physical inability to respond to extremes of temperature.

b. A comfortable climate can be maintained with heating or air conditioning; therefore, the degree of thermal stress is usually a function of socioeconomic factors.

c. The frail elderly and the obese are most vulnerable to heat exhaustion.

d. Mortality increases with age, temperature, and duration of the heat.

e. The frail elderly are also at the greatest risk of hypothermia.

f. Many communities have funds available to pay for heating and cooling for the elderly when necessary. This source of assistance should be considered.

B. Preventing illness and hospitalization

1. Screening and case-finding are important tools to prevent or control chronic disease processes before they threaten the quality of life and become more difficult and expensive to treat.

a. Screening programs have limitations.

b. Many elderly people do not have a regular physician and are lost to followup as workloads of health care teams increase.

c. Disability, isolation, and lack of income are both causes and effects of more serious problems.

d. House-to-house screening programs may be necessary to identify the needs of elders effectively.

2. Immunization against pneumonia and influenza decreases mortality in the elderly. Vaccines are widely available and are highly encouraged, especially for the frail elderly.
C. Hospitalization issues
1. Hospitalization is a major disruption of everyday life for both the patient and the family.
2. Medical disorders of the elderly may be better treated by addressing functional problems and limiting many tests and procedures that weaken the body and produce limited information.
3. Because of the efforts to control health care costs through DRGs, hospitals are pressured to discharge patients quickly, and many patients are sent home very ill.
4. Visiting nurses assist not only the client but also the family in understanding and complying with required treatment.
D. Institutionalization
1. *Institutionalization* refers to the placement of people who can no long care for themselves into a nursing home or care facility.
2. Only about 5% of the elderly population live in nursing homes, but the proportion increases rapidly with age, with more than 20% of those over the age of 85 living in institutions.
3. The median age of residents is 80, and the majority are widowed women.
4. Approximately 80% of all institutionalized elderly in the United States suffer from some type of mental disorder.
5. Institutionalization is usually the last resort when care of an aged relative has physically exhausted a family.
   a. Financial and emotional exhaustion may continue.
   b. Insurance policies for long-term care are available, but they are expensive.
   c. Medicare does not provide for institutionalization, and the issue of long-term care is of great concern to older people.
E. Death and bereavement
1. It is expected for people to experience the loss of parents, followed by loss of spouse, siblings, friends, and contemporaries, and culminating in one's own death.
2. Loss of adult children, who have themselves become aged, is now occurring.
3. The effects of bereavement in the elderly may continue for months and years.

4. Death as a crisis should include the concept of grief resolution as a process during which the survivor learns to live without a spouse.
   a. Assessment of past experience and coping skills used in adjusting to a previous loss and identification of support networks will assist in planning for care.
   b. Ministers, priests, rabbis, and other religious leaders have much experience in helping people through the grief process.
   c. Support groups for widows and widowers are often provided by religious organizations and are available for anyone in need.
F. Community environment
1. The need for mobility may necessitate driving a car when it is no longer safe.
2. The importance of mobility is recognized, and police are often sympathetic to elderly drivers, especially in small communities.
3. Widowed women living alone may have problems if they must maintain a house. Often they have never been employed and have difficulty in overseeing finances.
4. Many elderly have become poorer as fixed incomes fall behind inflation, and expenses, including expenses for health care, continue to rise.
G. Abuse of the elderly
1. Elder abuse is present in all parts of the United States.
2. It is less likely to be reported than child abuse, but public and professional awareness of the problem is growing with more frequent publicity.
3. Abusers are usually experiencing stress, possibly from alcoholism, drug addiction, marital problems, financial difficulty, or personality disorders.
4. Shame or fear makes elders unlikely to report abuse.
5. Abuse may be physical (physical restraining, beating, rape, and murder); psychological (isolation, threats, and fear); financial (theft of money or property); and neglect (not providing needed glasses, dentures, or clean clothes).
6. Most states have laws requiring mandatory reporting of elder abuse.
H. Crime and the elderly
1. Elders are easy targets for crime because of physical frailty and mental confusion.
2. Fear of robbery is common.
3. The major crime against the elderly is fraud.

4. Violent crimes are often found in older neighborhoods that have deteriorated.
5. The fear of being victimized is often enough to precipitate withdrawal, isolation, and depression.
6. To help deter crime, direct deposit of checks, including Social Security checks, into bank accounts is recommended. Transportation and a buddy system for shopping or social activities should be arranged.

I. Families of the elderly
1. Up to the age of 75, most elderly people do more for their children than their children do for them. When physical frailty becomes a problem, however, parent-child roles tend to become reversed and can be a major source of stress for all.
2. Daughters or daughters-in-law usually become the primary caregivers.
3. The quality of life for the frail elderly may be increased when care is given by a family member.
   a. There is a feeling of being wanted, comfort, and familiar surroundings and faces.
   b. There is more freedom and control than in an institution.
4. The physical and emotional costs of caring for the sick elder can be great for the caregiver.
   a. The caregiver is likely to report symptoms of depression, guilt, frustration and desperation.
   b. Alzheimer's disease is a major cause of caregiver stress.
5. The use of case management services for the elderly is a new and rapidly expanding industry.
   a. Services include the assessment and coordination of care for elders.
   b. These services are not usually covered by insurance but can bring great relief to over-stressed family members.
   c. Opportunities exist in this area for gerontological nurses.
   d. Case management programs provided by public and nonprofit agencies are available in many areas.

III. **Major Legislation**
A. The Social Security Act was originally passed in 1935 and has been amended 16 times.
   1. It is administered by agencies within the Department of Health and Human Services, including the Social Security Administration and Health Care Financing Administration.
   2. Most working people are enrolled automatically in the Social Security program, which is financed by contributions from employers, employees, and the self-employed.
   3. Social Security provides retirement benefits to people retiring at age 65, survivor's benefits for surviving children and widow(er)s, disability payments for people who are unable to work during the usual working years, and Medicare hospital insurance benefits.
   4. Part of each person's Social Security contribution is designated for Medicare, the national program of health insurance for the elderly. Medicare is divided in two parts.
      a. Part A is automatic, does not require contribution by the individual, and covers most of the cost of hospital care. The patient must pay a large deductible and copayments.
      b. Part B is medical insurance and requires a fee. It helps pay for physician services, outpatient services, and some other medical items. The monthly premium for part B was $46.10 in 1995 and usually increases each year.
   5. The elderly poor are eligible for Medicaid coverage.
   6. Managed care plans are becoming widely encouraged for elders.
B. The Older Americans Act established the Administration on Aging in 1965.
   1. Its purpose is to identify the needs, concerns and interests of older people and to coordinate available federal resources to meet those needs.
   2. The act was amended in 1973 to provide local planning of programs. The programs must include nutrition services such as home-delivered meals or meals provided in communal settings.
   3. Throughout the country, senior centers are sites for nutrition programs; recreational, social, and health programs; housing assistance; counseling; and information.
C. The Research on Aging Act created the National Institute on Aging within the National Institutes of Health in 1974.
   1. Its purpose is to conduct and support biomedical, social, and behavioral research and training related to the aging process and the diseases and other special problems and needs of the aged.
   2. Health promotion, functional independence, and quality of life are research goals.

3. The National Institute on Aging is a source of funding for nurses interested in researching problems on aging.
D. The Age Discrimination in Employment Act (1967) provides workers ages 40- 65 with the same opportunities as younger employees for participation in employee benefit plans.
E. The Employee Retirement Income Security Act (1974) was passed to safeguard employee pension plans.
F. The Retirement Equity Act (1984) increased protection for surviving spouses of pension-eligible workers.

IV. **New Concepts of Community Care**—Across the United States, new ways to meet the needs of the elderly are being devised. Four are described here.
A. Nursing home as senior center
1. In some areas, there are programs intended to give nursing homes greater visibility and deeper roots in the community and to provide extended programs for the well elderly.
2. This model provides a meeting place and opportunity for social activities and networking.
3. Transportation may be arranged for members who need assistance, and meals may be provided.
B. Generations Together
1. Generations Together is a program that works to use strengths of one age group to meet the needs of another age group in reciprocal relationships.
2. Activities include intergenerational theater, literature discussions, and education of the homebound elderly.
C. Mutual assistance: The elder helping the elderly
1. In many areas, churches group together to combine resources and address social problems.
2. Some programs promote and encourage independence of elders by establishing a neighborhood network of volunteers to provide mutual assistance, information, and services. Services may include nutrition, transportation, health education, caregiver support and respite, increased social contact, counseling, home maintenance assistance, and referral.
D. Social-health maintenance organization demonstration
1. This is a research demonstration project to study the feasibility of providing the elderly with a single prepaid program of pre-

ventive, acute, and long-term services by integrating community-based care into the HMO model.
2. This project provides information for policy and practice in decision-making to encourage efficient, effective healthcare for elders.

V. **Application of the Nursing Process**—A theory base applicable to the client's needs should provide a framework within which the nursing process is used. A number of theories related to aging have been described in literature and may be applicable to planning appropriate care for elderly clients.
A. Selected social theories of aging
1. Activity theory—Maintenance of optimal levels of activity from the middle years of life is a key to successful aging.
2. Disengagement theory—As people age, their needs change from active involvement to withdrawal and impending death. In addition to withdrawal of the individual from society, there is the withdrawal of society from the aged.
3. Loss of major life roles theory—This theory claims that disengagement is forced by denying older people society roles. This led to establishment of government programs to provide volunteer and work opportunities.
4. Continuity theory—An individual's unique personality and behavioral characteristics and habits continue into old age.
5. Socially disruptive events theory—If life is severely disrupted in a number of ways in a brief period of time, social withdrawal becomes an appropriate response.
6. Reconstruction theory—Negative labeling of the elderly by society may lead to a view of the elderly as incompetent and helpless.
7. Age stratification theory—Societies are inevitably stratified by age and class. Inequality of the elderly depends on their life course experiences and is due to physical and mental changes that take place and the history of the time through which they have lived.
8. Modernization theory—Loss of social status among the aged is universal in cultures in which modernization is occurring.
B. Assessment
1. Data collection should be complete and systematic.
a. A standardized form used by the agency is helpful, but the nurse should adapt it to situations outside the norm.

b. The nurse can use systems theory, focusing on the client as the system, where the client's biological, psychological, and social subsystems may be examined.

c. The client's suprasystems, such as family interaction and neighborhood, should also be assessed.

d. The nurse can choose to use the epidemiological approach; in this approach, the client is the host, a problem is the agent, and the environment includes all causes of and possible solutions for the problem.

2. Data collected must take into account aging changes and must be measured against elderly norms.

3. Assessment categories should include nutrition, elimination, activity, medication consumption, body protection, cognitive tasks, life changes and the environment.

4. Assessment of the family and community of a client follows the same systematic data collection methods.

C. Planning

1. Planning for intervention should be theory-based.

2. The nurse should set short- and long-term goals that are congruent with the desired outcomes of the client.

3. Compliance will often not be good unless the patient sees some value in the outcomes.

D. Evaluation

1. Evaluation is a joint activity of the client and the nurse.

2. Evaluation measures movement toward or away from a specified goal and gives dynamic feedback that affects planning and intervention.

3. Many chronic illnesses have a long time-frame; because of this, the standard for evaluation may be prevention of deterioration rather than cure of a disease.

VI. **Allocation of Resources for Senior Health**

A. The increasing number of older people needing health care is stimulating discussion on the kind of services that should be provided.

B. Currently, four themes exist concerning ethical decision-making in an aging society.

1. Autonomy versus beneficence (the rights, wishes, and competency of a client to accept or refuse help)

2. Issues of death, dying, and termination of treatment

3. Allocation of resources in an aging population

4. Family caregiving and/or the obligation to provide care.

VII. **Research on the Health of the Elderly**

A. Studies on the elderly and the process of aging are needed in all areas.

B. Several specific areas are particularly in need of study.

1. The action of medications in older people

2. Drug dosage and frequency

3. Causes of different rates of physical and mental aging

4. Predicting and planning for the welfare of the majority while allowing flexibility for the needs of others.

VIII. **Roles of the Community Health Nurse**

A. The community health nurse should be a resource person, client advocate, health educator, case manager, facilitator, coordinator of care between agencies, researcher, and care provider.

B. Nurses should also seek leadership in organizations that affect their clients and should be political lobbyists.

TEACHING STRATEGIES

1. Invite a geriatric nurse practitioner to speak to the class about working with elderly clients. Have the nurse discuss specific needs of elders and ways to work with them effectively.

2. Encourage a class discussion of personal experiences in helping care for elderly family members. Discuss specific physical, psychological, social, spiritual, and economic needs. How were problems resolved? What resources were used? What are some ethical problems that have been encountered?

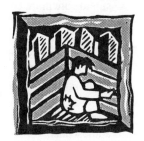

CHAPTER 15

The Homeless

ANNOTATED LEARNING OBJECTIVES

1. Discuss two meanings of the term homeless.

The term *homeless* refers to an individual who lacks a fixed, regular, and adequate night-time residence and/or whose primary night-time residence is a supervised publicly or privately operated shelter, an institution that provides a temporary residence, or a public or private place not ordinarily used for sleeping, such as a car or garage.

2. Describe the scope of homelessness in the United States.

The Census Bureau has attempted to count the homeless population and has identified approximately 237,000 people (counting only those in emergency shelters, streets, and shelters for abused women). Single men account for almost half of the homeless; families with children account for 39%; 11% are single women; and 3% are unaccompanied minors. Ethnically, 53% are black, 31% are white, 1% are Hispanic, 3% are Native American, and 1% are Asian.

The numbers of homeless people appear to have increased dramatically during the 1980s. Based on lifetime prevalence estimates, about 13.5 million adults (7.4%) have been homeless during some point in their lives.

3. Analyze factors that contribute to homelessness.

The factors that contribute to homelessness are complex and varied. They include poverty; changes in the labor market (shift of goods production to services, labor market that demands an educated workforce, etc.); lack of affordable housing; deinstitutionalization of the mentally ill; and heavy use of alcohol and illicit drugs (particularly crack cocaine).

4. Identify major health problems among various homeless aggregates.

Health problems vary considerably among different aggregates. Some of the more common problems are listed below.

Homeless men—Homeless men experience acute physical health problems, respiratory infections, trauma, and skin disorders at higher rates than men in the general population. Chronic disorders (hypertension, gastrointestinal problems, peripheral vascular disease, chronic obstructive pulmonary disease, and seizure disorders) are more prevalent among homeless populations. AIDS, tuberculosis, and STDs occur at higher rates than in the general population. Many of these conditions are exacerbated by alcoholism, which occurs more frequently among the homeless.

Homeless women—Homeless women suffer more acute and chronic health problems than the general population. STDs are common among homeless women. The pregnancy rate among homeless women is surprisingly high: approximately 10% of homeless women were pregnant compared to 7% of the general population. Approximately 34% of homeless women meet criteria for post-traumatic stress syndrome. Approximately 20% abuse alcohol, and 10–20% suffer from drug problems. A history of childhood physical and sexual abuse and assault is common.

Homeless children—Because homeless women frequently lack prenatal care and sufficient nutrition, they are more likely to deliver low-birthweight infants. Infant mortality rates are higher for homeless women. Homeless children have immunization delays, upper respiratory tract and ear infections, asthma, skin disorders, diarrhea, and anemia more often than housed poor children. More homeless children lack sufficient food. Depression and anxiety occur more often among homeless children, and homeless children are more likely to lack personal and social skills. Language and gross and fine motor skills tend to be delayed.

Homeless adolescents—Unintended pregnancy, STDs, alcohol and drug abuse, depression, and suicide are more common among homeless adolescents. Physical and sexual abuse, skin disorders, anemia, drug and alcohol abuse, and unintentional injuries occur more often among homeless adolescents than in adolescents in the general population. Depression, suicide ideation, and behavior disorders are more common. There is a higher rate of negative pregnancy outcomes than in non-homeless adolescents.

Homeless families—Homeless families are predominantly female-headed households, and the children are usually preschoolers. Relationships that homeless mothers typically have had with men are characterized by instability, conflict, and violence. Many of the male partners are substance abusers.

Homeless people with mental health and substance use problems—Approximately 59% of the homeless population have a diagnosed mental illness. Approximately 50% of homeless men and 15% of homeless women are alcoholics. Between 10 and 20% of homeless single adults suffer from a psychiatric disorder, substance abuse, or co-morbidity. The homeless population experiences depression at a higher rate than the general population.

5. *Discuss access to health care for the homeless.*

Multiple complex factors reduce access to health care for the homeless. Access to the health care system includes the general components of availability, accessibility, accommodation, affordability, and acceptability. The homeless cannot produce the documentation of residency necessary to qualify for many services. Lack of storage and personal papers contribute to this problem. Problems with distance and transportation, lack of a permanent mailing address, and lack of money are additional barriers to access.

6. *Analyze the health problems of the homeless using upstream thinking and a social justice perspective.*

Market justice is the dominant model in the United States; it states that people are entitled to valued ends such as status, income, happiness according to their own individual efforts. Market justice stresses individual responsibility, minimal collective action, and freedom from collective obligations. Market justice contributes to a "downstream approach" to dealing with social problems such as

homelessness because it holds individuals responsible for their own condition and negates the responsibility of society to share in prevention.

Social justice promotes a position that all people are entitled to key ends such as access to health care and minimum standards of income, and all members must accept the collective burden to provide for a fair distribution of these ends. Social justice supports the "upstream approach" to addressing the problem of homelessness. In this model, efforts focus on what contributes to homelessness, such as substance abuse and lack of access to affordable housing, education, and employment.

7. *Apply knowledge about the homeless when planning community health services for this aggregate.*

Nurses may have contact with homeless people in a variety of settings, including schools, jails, emergency rooms, community clinics, and shelters. Efforts to address the health and social needs of the homeless should follow the nursing process and should be planned at the individual, family, and aggregate levels. Considering all levels of prevention is essential.

LECTURE OUTLINE

I. **Definitions and Prevalence of Homelessness**
  A. The definition of the term *homeless* includes individuals who meet the following criteria.
    1. Lacks a fixed, regular, adequate night-time residence
    2. Has a primary night-time residence that is a supervised publicly or privately operated shelter (welfare hotel, shelter, transitional housing)
    3. Has a primary residence that is a temporary residence for individuals that are intended to be institutionalized
    4. Sleeps in a public or private place not ordinarily used for sleeping, such as a car, garage, or park bench
    5. Lives temporarily with a family member or friend
  B. Demographic data
    1. The Census Bureau has attempted to count the homeless population and has identified approximately 237,000 people, counting only those in emergency shelters, streets, and shelters for abused women.
    2. Single men account for almost half of the homeless population; families with children account for 39%; single women 11%; unaccompanied minors 3%.

3. Ethnically, 53% of the homeless population is black; 31% is white; 1% is Hispanic; 3% are Native American; and 1% are Asian.

II. Factors That Contribute to Homelessness

A. Poverty—14.5% of the population is classified as "poor."

B. Changes in the labor market decrease job opportunities and create poverty.
   1. Shift from production of goods to services
   2. Labor market that demands an educated work force

C. Lack of affordable housing—The cost of housing rose during the 1970s and 1980s, increasing the need for public subsidized housing dramatically.

D. Deinstitutionalization of the mentally ill
   1. Approximately one-fourth of the homeless population has a history of mental illness.
   2. The limitation of beds in psychiatric facilities, end of involuntary commitment, and federal cutbacks for community mental health have created a context in which individuals with mental illness are at risk of becoming homeless.

E. Heavy use of alcohol and illicit drugs (particularly crack cocaine)

III. Health Status of the Homeless

A. Homeless men
   1. Homeless men experience acute physical health problems, respiratory infections, trauma, and skin disorders at higher rates than men in the general population.
   2. Chronic disorders such as hypertension, gastrointestinal problems, peripheral vascular disease, chronic obstructive pulmonary disease, and seizure disorders are more prevalent among homeless populations.
   3. AIDS, tuberculosis, and STDs occur at higher rates than in the general population.
   4. Many health conditions are exacerbated by alcoholism, which is the most common illness among the homeless.
   5. Homeless men are more likely to be unemployed or under-employed or to be military veterans than men in the general population.

B. Homeless women
   1. Homeless women suffer more acute and chronic health problems than the general population.
   2. STDs are more than twice as common among the homeless.
   3. Pregnancy rates among homeless women are surprisingly high: approximately 10% of homeless women are pregnant, compared to 7% of women in the general population.
   4. Homelessness affects a woman's sense of identity and her feelings of self-worth and self-sufficiency.
   5. Approximately 34% of homeless women meet criteria for post-traumatic stress syndrome.
   6. Approximately 20% abuse alcohol, and 10–20% suffer from drug problems.
   7. A history of childhood physical and sexual abuse and assault is common.
   8. Many homeless women have limited education and job opportunities and fragmented support networks.

C. Homeless children
   1. Because homeless women frequently lack prenatal care and sufficient nutrition, they are more likely to deliver low-birthweight infants.
   2. Infant mortality rates are higher for infants born to homeless women.
   3. Homeless children have more immunization delays, upper respiratory tract and ear infections, asthma, skin disorders, diarrhea, and anemia than housed poor children.
   4. Many homeless children suffer from lack of sufficient food.
   5. Depression and anxiety occur more often among homeless children.
   6. Homeless children are more likely than other children to lack personal, social, and language skills. Gross and fine motor skills are often delayed.
   7. Homeless children miss more days of school than other children and are more likely to repeat grades.

D. Homeless adolescents
   1. Homeless adolescents face serious health problems such as unintended pregnancy, STDs, and alcohol and drug abuse.
   2. Physical and sexual abuse, skin disorders, anemia, and unintentional injuries are more common in homeless adolescents than in adolescents in the general population.
   3. Depression, suicide ideation, and behavior disorders are common among homeless adolescents.
   4. Homeless adolescent females have a higher rate of negative pregnancy outcomes than housed females.
   5. Runaway or homeless adolescents, both male and female, constitute a large percentage of youth involved in prostitution.

E.   Homeless families
1. There are four types of homeless families.
   a. Unemployed couples
   b. Mothers who have left relationships
   c. AFDC mothers
   d. Mothers who are homeless teenagers
2. Homeless families are predominantly female-headed households, and the children are usually preschoolers.
3. Homeless mothers typically have had relationships with men that are characterized by instability, conflict, and violence. Many of the male partners are substance abusers.

F. Homeless people with mental health or substance use problems
1. Approximately 59% of the homeless have a diagnosed mental illness.
2. Approximately 50% of homeless men and 15% of homeless women are alcoholics.
3. Between 10 and 20% of homeless single adults suffer from a psychiatric disorder, substance use, or co-morbidity.
4. For some, mental illness and substance use cause homelessness; for others, mental illness or substance abuse is the result of homelessness.
5. Beginning in the 1960s, deinstitutionalization made it difficult to commit an individual to a psychiatric facility involuntarily, and many of those who would have been retained in a mental hospital are among the homeless.
6. Homeless people experience clinical depression at a higher rate than the general population.

IV. Health Care Access for the Homeless Population
A. Access to the health care system includes five general components.
1. *Availability*—the relationship of the amount (or number of providers and facilities) and type of health care services to the amount and type of client needs
2. *Accessibility*—the relationship of the location of the services to the client's location
3. *Accommodation*—the relationship of the organization of services (hours of operation, appointment systems) to the client's ability to accommodate them.
4. *Affordability*—the relationship of the price of services or payment requirements and the client's ability to pay
5. *Acceptability*—the relationship of client attitudes about providers and provider attitudes about acceptable client characteristics.

B. Barriers to access
1. The homeless cannot produce the documentation of residency necessary to qualify for many services. Lack of storage and personal papers contribute to this problem.
2. Problems with distance and transportation, lack of a permanent mailing address, and lack of money are additional barriers to access.

V. Conceptual Approaches to Health Care for the Homeless Population
A. Market justice
1. Market justice states that people are entitled to valued ends such as status, income, and happiness according to their own individual efforts.
2. Market justice stresses individual responsibility, minimal collective action, and freedom from collective obligations.
3. The market justice model is a "downstream approach" to dealing with social problems of the homeless because it holds individuals responsible for their own condition and negates the responsibility of society to share in prevention.
4. Market justice is the dominant model in the United States.

B. Social justice
1. Social justice states that all people are entitled to key ends such as access to health care and minimum standards of income, and that all members must accept collective burdens to provide for a fair distribution of these ends.
2. Social justice supports the "upstream approach" to address the problems of homelessness.
3. In the social justice model, efforts focus on what contributes to homelessness.
   a. Lack of access to affordable housing
   b. Lack of education
   c. Lack of employment
   d. Substance abuse

VI. Application of the Nursing Process
A. Nurses may have contact with homeless people in a variety of settings: schools, jails, emergency rooms, community clinics, and shelters.
B. Efforts to address the health and social needs should follow the nursing process and be directed to the individual, family, and aggregate levels.
C. Consideration of all levels of prevention is essential.

VII. Research and the Homeless

A. Research on the homeless is limited for a number of reasons.

1. The transient nature of homelessness makes it difficult to locate and maintain study participants.

2. Alcoholism, mental illness, and other acute and chronic conditions can impede data collection.

3. Language and cultural differences, problems with literacy, and reluctance on the part of the homeless may also contribute to difficulties in conducting research in this population.

B. More research into providing a better understanding of the complex problems facing the homeless is encouraged.

C. Qualitative research should be conducted to understand personal and social factors that contribute to homelessness and how people's lives are affected by homelessness.

D. An interdisciplinary focus should be maintained to address the complex causes of homelessness and to determine appropriate, effective interventions.

TEACHING STRATEGIES

1. Invite a health care professional who works with the homeless (preferably a nurse) to speak to the class about issues surrounding homelessness.

2. Have students do a "community assessment" of the homeless population in their city or town. Students should explore census and vital statistics data where available; talk with employees and volunteers from local community resource organizations; and conduct a "windshield assessment" of areas where groups of homeless people "live."

3. If the group is small enough, arrange for a visit to a homeless shelter. Identify potential projects students might develop to help meet the needs of homeless individuals, families, and groups.

CHAPTER 16

Rural Health

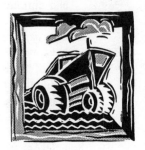

ANNOTATED LEARNING OBJECTIVES

1. *Discuss the definitions of the term* **rural.**

The U.S. Census Bureau classifies as *rural* those people who live in towns with a population of less than 2500 or in open country. The Census Bureau further divides the rural population into *farm* and *nonfarm.* A county that contains an urban population center of 50,000 or more people is considered a *metropolitan* county, and all other counties are designated as *nonmetropolitan.* The term *frontier* refers to an area with a population density of less than six people per square mile.

2. *Explain why rural populations and geographic areas must be defined as appropriately as possible.*

The concept of rurality encompasses several factors, including population density, types of employment, and cultural diversity. There is great variability in rural regions throughout the United States. Rural populations differ because of a complex mix of geographic, social, and economic factors. As a result, health care planners and health care professionals should remember that there are many "rural Americas in rural America."

3. *Describe features of the health care system and population characteristics common to the rural aggregate.*

Residents of rural communities have health patterns and problems related to demographic and geographic patterns (i.e., age, gender, occupation, race/ethnicity, availability of health information, preventive and illness services, sewage and water systems, and transportation). Age is a particularly important consideration in planning health care for rural communities. The elderly often live at or near the poverty level in most rural regions; they tend to

be isolated and lack access to health care. They are increasingly the primary caregivers for spouses or parents. In western states, fetal, infant, and maternal mortality are somewhat higher in nonmetropolitan areas, and care in later prenatal stages is problematic.

4. *Identify structural barriers to health care.*

Barriers to health care among rural residents include lower income levels, higher unemployment, and higher poverty rates than urban dwellers. Employment often does not include insurance coverage in industries such as agriculture, forestry, and fishing. Structural barriers to adequate health care include availability of services, distance, isolation, low population density, and lack of transportation. These factors contribute to lack of availability of health care services and lack of access to services that do exist.

5. *Describe factors that place farmers and farm families at risk for accidents.*

Farmers and their families are at risk for accidents due to several causes. Agricultural machinery is the most common cause of both fatal and nonfatal injuries, and tractors pose the greatest threat. Highly variable environmental conditions (temperature extremes, storms) are associated with increased frequency of accidents. Farmers are located in isolated areas and often work alone. This places them at greater risk when an accident occurs, because farmers are less likely to have timely access to emergency or trauma care compared to people living in nonrural settings.

6. *Describe the importance of the informal care network to rural health and social services.*

Limited availability and accessibility of formal health care resources, combined with self-reliance and self-help of rural residents, have resulted in the development of strong informal care and social support networks in rural communities. Informal care networks include people in the community who have assumed positions of "caregiver" by their life situations, social roles, or individual qualities. They often provide support in the form of direct care, advice, or information. Family members, friends, and neighbors may be informal providers of care. Professional health care providers must recognize the strengths and contributions of the informal care system and use them as a community resource.

7. *Describe the unique features of rural community health nursing practice.*

Rural nursing is the diagnosis and treatment of a diverse population consisting of people of all ages, with a variety of human responses to actual and potential occupational hazards and actual or potential health problems. Rural nurses practice professional nursing within the physical and sociocultural context of sparsely populated communities, including aspects of maternity, pediatric, medical/surgical, and emergency nursing.

In rural community health nursing, the nurse must meet the health needs of smaller populations distributed over a larger geographical area. Few resources are available compared with those found in urban settings. The rural community health nurse has greater autonomy in making decisions to provide comprehensive care. Practice settings for rural community health nurses include the county health department, primary care physician offices, community health centers, and home health agencies.

8. *Apply upstream perspective to health promotion, prevention of illness, and premature death and disability.*

Upstream thinking focuses the community health nurse toward seeking an understanding of the precursors of poor health within a designated population. In rural settings, nurses can assist in identifying and remediating actual and potential health threats. Nurses can also assist by helping the community recognize health problems and direct them in social action to address health problems. In rural settings, the community health nurse provides for optimal health through primary health care and health promotion.

LECTURE OUTLINE

I. **Rural United States**
A. Almost 25% of Americans live in rural areas.

1. This includes about 26% of the children and elderly and 50% of the nation's poor.
2. Fewer than 10% of rural dwellers are farmers.
3. Traditional nonfarm rural occupations include mining, government employment, and manufacturing.

B. Definitions of rural population
1. The concept of rurality encompasses several factors, including population density, types of employment, and cultural diversity.
2. There is great variability in rural regions throughout the United States.
3. The U.S. Census Bureau classifies those people who live in towns with a population of less than 2500 or open country as *rural,* and further divides them into *farm* and *nonfarm* populations. The term *frontier* refers to an area with a population density of less than six people per square mile.
4. A county that contains an urban population center of 50,000 or more people is considered a *metropolitan* county, and all other counties are designated as *nonmetropolitan.* About two-thirds of American counties are nonmetropolitan.
5. Rural populations differ from one another due to a complex mix of geographic, social, and economic factors, and health care planners and health care professionals should remember that there are many "rural Americas in rural America."

II. **Community and Statistical Indicators of Rural Health**
A. Rural communities vary considerably based on economic and cultural resources, employment patterns, population density, relative isolation, age distribution and ethnic composition.
1. There are differences in factors such as education, employment, income, health, and lifestyle patterns when compared with urban populations.
2. Infant mortality is slightly higher, and accidental deaths are significantly higher in rural areas.
3. Rural residents are more likely to be obese, smoke heavily, and consume more alcohol than urban dwellers. In addition, they are far more likely to be exposed to occupational hazards.
B. Barriers to health care—Rural residents face a number of barriers to health care when compared to urban dwellers.

1. Rural residents typically have lower income levels, higher unemployment, and higher poverty rates.
2. Employment in industries such as agriculture, forestry, and fishing often does not include insurance coverage.
3. Rural groups have problems obtaining health care due to structural, financial, and personal barriers to accessing health care services.
4. Availability of services, distance, isolation, lack of transportation, and low population density all contribute to lack of availability of health care services, as well as lack of access to services that do exist.

C. Structural, financial, and personal factors and health status
   1. Rural populations have health patterns and problems related to demographic and geographic patterns
      a. Age
      b. Gender
      c. Occupation
      d. Race/ethnicity
      e. Availability of health information
      f. Availability of preventive and illness services
      g. Sewage and water systems
      h. Transportation
   2. Age is an important consideration in planning health care for rural communities.
      a. The elderly often live at or near the poverty level in most rural regions.
      b. The elderly tend to be isolated and lack access to health care.
      c. They are increasingly the primary caregivers for spouses or parents.
   3. In western states, fetal, infant and maternal mortality rates are somewhat higher in nonmetropolitan areas, and care in later prenatal stages is problematic.
   4. Substance use and abuse by young people in rural American is of concern. Smokeless tobacco and alcohol are particularly problematic.
   5. Disabling injuries and mortality related to occupation are dramatically higher in rural populations.
      a. Mechanical, chemical, and thermal injuries, as well as psychological stress with higher suicide rates, are found in farmers.
      b. Miners and loggers work in hazardous conditions and suffer from a variety of acute and chronic problems.

6. Rural adults participate in preventive behaviors less often and have less contact with physicians than residents of urban areas.
7. Rural populations more often suffer from conditions associated with poor sanitation and overcrowding, pesticide exposure, and problems related to pregnancy and early childhood.

III. **Specific Rural Aggregates—Agricultural Workers**
A. Agriculture has a significant impact on the health status of most rural communities.
   1. The health risks of farming are different, rather than fewer, than risks encountered in metropolitan areas.
   2. Agriculture, construction and mining share the highest rates of worker fatality of all U.S. industries.
   3. Farmers and their families have been found to have excess risk for conditions associated with hearing loss, respiratory illness, nonfatal accidents, and chemical hazards.
B. Accidents and injuries
   1. Highly variable environmental conditions such as temperature extremes are associated with increased frequency of accidents.
   2. Farmers are located in isolated areas and often work alone.
      a. Their location and working conditions place them at greater risk for injury.
      b. When an accident occurs, farmers are less likely to have timely access to emergency or trauma care compared with people living in non-rural settings.
   3. Agricultural machinery is the most common cause of both fatal and non-fatal injuries, with tractors posing the greatest threat.
C. Acute and chronic illnesses
   1. Both acute and chronic respiratory illnesses occur frequently in farmers.
   2. This is due in part to chronic exposure to grain dusts, fungi, or toxic gases such as pesticides.
   3. Rural community health nurses should be aware of signs and symptoms of acute pesticide poisoning.
      a. Headache
      b. Dizziness
      c. Diaphoresis
      d. Nausea and vomiting
   4. If untreated, affected people may experience a progression of symptoms, including dyspnea, bronchospasm, and muscle twitching. Deaths, although not common, do occur.

D. Migrant and seasonal farm workers
   1. Each year, an estimated 3 million farm workers participate in crop planting, weeding, and harvesting activities throughout the United States.
   2. Most migrant farm workers are Mexican or Mexican-American.
   3. The migrant and seasonal farm workers are a very vulnerable population due to numerous health risks, low income, and migratory status.
   4. They often experience physical and cultural isolation.
   5. Sensitivity to cultural beliefs and lifestyles can aid in planning and implementing care to meet the health needs of these aggregates.

IV. **Application of Theories and "Thinking Upstream" Concepts to Rural Health**
   A. Attack community-based problems at their roots
      1. Upstream thinking focuses the community health nurse on seeking an understanding of the precursors of poor health within a designated population.
      2. In rural settings, nurses can help identify and remedy actual and potential health threats.
      3. Nurses can also help the community recognize health problems and health threats; they can then help direct social action to address these problems.
   B. Emphasize the "doing" aspects of health
      1. Rural residents often equate the functioning and performance of daily activities with health. Being able "to do" is highly valued.
      2. Active involvement of the population is key to achieving success in program planning and implementation.
      3. This perspective may be helpful in health-related teaching.
   C. Maximize the use of informal networks
      1. Recognizing informal networks and using them to implement programs and change is essential.
      2. The involvement of community leaders in change is vitally important.
      3. Strategies will rarely be successful without maximizing the investment of community constituencies in their own well-being.

V. **Rural Health Care Delivery System**
   A. Rural health care statistics
      1. It is thought that about 10 million rural dwellers (15%) are without a regular source of health care and that an additional 16 million (21%) live in communities without adequate primary care providers.
      2. Unfortunately, rural health care has been modeled after urban health care (specialist providers, hospital-based, acute care and high-tech, expensive procedures).
      3. In the 1970s and 1980s, many rural health initiatives were directed at making hospitals financially viable and the center of caring for the community's health.
      4. During the late 1980s and early 1990s, hospitals in rural areas developed an enhanced health promotion and prevention emphasis for community members to help address philosophic differences between providers of health care and providers of illness care.
   B. Alternative Facility Model
      1. In the late 1980s and early 1990s, almost 200 rural hospitals closed nationally.
      2. People in frontier counties have significant problems finding primary health care.
      3. In the United States, 11% of rural hospitals are in frontier areas. These hospitals serve approximately 46% of the U.S. land area, in which 1% of the population resides.
      4. To improve access to health care, new rural hospital models such as the Alternative Facility Model are being developed, often using nurse practitioners or physician assistants as primary care providers.
   C. Health care provider shortages
      1. The shortage of health care professionals is a barrier to health care delivery.
      2. The ratio of nurses to population in rural areas is less than half that of urban areas (319 vs. 725 RNs per 10,000).
      3. Although approximately 25% of the population lives in nonmetropolitan counties, only 13% of physicians and 8.7% of nurses practice in those counties.
      4. The supply of physician assistants and nurse practitioners has not kept up with need for their services in rural areas.
   D. Community-wide health care system
      1. To cope with limited facilities and providers, rural health care planners recommend development of a community-wide health care system, with the hospital as one component.
      2. The focus of this system is community-based care in the form of community-oriented primary care services (COPC).
   E. Primary care and primary health care
      1. *Primary care* refers to care provided in an office or clinic setting by a provider such

as a physician, nurse, nurse practitioner, physician assistant, mental health counselor, or other health care professional who takes responsibility for the client's health.

2. COPC is often called *primary health care,* meaning that providers address the health and illness concerns not just of the group of clients they see in the clinic/office, but of the community as a whole, using an epidemiological orientation.

3. The providers integrate components of public health, health promotion, and disease prevention into primary care practice.

4. Community health nurses can use their knowledge of community assessment, aggregates, and community involvement to assist in the planning process or organizing community-based care.

VI. **Community-Based Care**—*Community-based care* often refers to services including home health care, in-home hospice care, nutrition programs, community mental health, and adult day care. Community participation also involves decision-making about health care services.

A. Home care and hospice programs
1. In rural areas and frontier areas, home care and hospice programs are often contracted through larger regional agencies.
2. A larger agency may hire a nurse from the area to provide home health care or hospice services in that area.
3. Nurse case management and development of local resources are helpful in providing information and a network of providers.

B. Rural mental health care
1. Although little information is available on the prevalence or types of mental illnesses specifically found in rural areas, large sections of rural populations are believed to be at risk for illness and are without mental health care.
2. Lack of awareness and acceptance of mental health care providers are major barriers for mental health care professionals practicing in rural areas.
3. Problems recognized by mental health providers include more diverse practice, fewer opportunities for ongoing education, and fewer professionals for consultations, compared to their colleagues in urban settings.

C. Emergency services
1. Emergency medical services (EMS) have become increasingly important in rural areas as many rural hospitals close.

2. Often small communities have a volunteer EMS response team but no local hospital or medical clinic.
3. Rural EMS teams cover sparsely populated geographic areas.
4. EMS systems are important in decreasing the morbidity and mortality of rural people needing emergency care.
5. Shortage of volunteers, lower level of training, curricula that often do not reflect rural needs, lack of guidance from physicians, and lack of physician orientation to the EMS system, contribute to problems with rural EMS systems.

D. Informal care systems
1. Limited availability and accessibility of formal health care resources, combined with the self-reliance and self-help of rural residents, have resulted in the development of strong informal care and social support networks in rural communities.
2. Informal care networks include people in the community who have assumed positions of caregivers because of their life situations, social roles, or individual qualities.
3. They often provide support in the form of direct care, advice, or information.
4. Family members, friends, and neighbors may be informal providers of care.
5. Professional health care providers must recognize the strengths and contributions of the informal care system and use them as a community resource.

E. Rural public health departments
1. Less than 40% of Americans are currently served by a local health department that performs the traditional public health functions of assessment, policy development, and health assurance.
2. Many rural counties are too small to support a health department staffed by trained personnel or have insufficient financial resources to support the needed services. Thus, many small rural health departments can offer only programs funded by federal programs.

F. Managed care in the rural environment
1. In rural areas, the expansion of managed care is progressing through development of health care delivery networks with managed care elements.
2. The National Rural Health Association has identified potential benefits and risks of managed care in rural areas.

a. Benefits include the potential to lower primary care costs, improve the quality of care, and help stabilize the local rural health care system.

b. Possible risks include high start-up and administrative costs, and concerns regarding the effect of the presence of large, urban-based, for-profit managed care companies on the community's health.

VII. Legislation and Programs Affecting Public Health

A. History of health legislation pertaining to rural areas

1. In 1922, the Sheppard-Towner Act was passed to address health issues related to mother/child care in rural areas. This act provided federal funding for personal health services and shifted public health from disease prevention to promotion of overall health.

2. During the 1960s, block grants for public health programs became the primary source of funding for rural health programs.

3. The Social Security Act (1935) provided financing for training of public health personnel and addressing public health problems. The Social Security Amendments of 1965 created direct federal aid to individuals through Medicare and Medicaid.

B. Current health care programs affecting rural areas

1. Health care programs that affect the availability and provision of health care services in rural areas

a. Federally sponsored programs such as Medicare, Medicaid, Department of Veterans Affairs, and Indian Health Services

b. Federal block grants to the states, which provide funding for maternal/child health services, preventive health programs, mental health programs, and alcohol and drug abuse programs

c. Programs that augment the health resources available to underserved areas through the Department of Health and Human Services or the Health Resources and Services Administration

2. Programs that augment health personnel

a. The National Health Service Corps (NHSC) and the Area Health Education Centers encourage health professionals to practice in health personnel shortage areas through volunteer, scholarship, and loan repayment programs.

b. Special programs also support advanced practice nurses and minority and disadvantaged students preparing for health professions careers.

3. Programs that augment health care facilities and services

a. The community health centers program (administered by the Health Resources and Services Administration) benefits underserved areas and populations by providing primary health care for rural people.

b. The Migrant Health Centers program provides services for migrant and seasonal farm workers and their families.

4. Programs that assist with health care policy planning and research—The Office of Rural Health Policy advises providers and planners on rural health issues such as availability and access to health professionals and prioritization and financing of rural health care services. It also manages the Rural Health Research Center grant program.

VIII. Rural Community Health Nursing

A. Characteristics of rural nursing

1. Rural nursing applies professional nursing to the physical and sociocultural context of sparsely populated communities.

2. Rural nursing is the diagnosis and treatment of a diversified population of people of all ages and a variety of human responses to actual or potential occupational hazards, and/or actual or potential health problems.

3. Services may include prenatal care, infant and child care, home care for acute and chronic disease, hospice care, school health, and mental health.

4. Rural nursing combines aspects of maternity, pediatric, medical/surgical, and emergency nursing within a given rural area.

5. In rural community health nursing, the nurse must meet the health needs of smaller populations distributed over a larger geographical area.

6. Few resources are available compared with those found in urban settings.

7. The rural community health nurse has greater autonomy in making decisions to provide comprehensive care.

8. Practice settings for rural community health nurses include county health departments,

primary care physician offices, community health centers, and home health agencies.

9. The nurse often functions independently, applying the nursing process in promoting and preserving health for rural aggregates.

B. Nursing roles in community health practice
1. The practice of community health nursing in rural communities is broad-based and generalist in nature.
2. Rural nurses need good decision-making skills to practice in settings where there may be little professional support and supervision.
3. Nursing roles include educator, direct care provider, case manager, coordinator, and administrator.

C. Advantages and disadvantages of rural nursing
1. Rural community health nursing is both rewarding and challenging.
2. Positive aspects of rural nursing practice are autonomy, professional status, and feeling of being valued by the community.
3. Disadvantages include physical and professional isolation, problems related to scarce resources (low salary, fewer positions), various problems within the work environment, role diffusion, and lack of anonymity.

IX. **Application of the Nursing Process**
A. Assessment
1. Assessing the health care needs of rural populations requires collaboration with other disciplines and community leaders.
2. The assessment should identify individuals, families, and aggregates at risk of illness, disability, or premature death and should include an assessment of the community's ability to meet its health responsibilities.

B. Diagnosis—Diagnosis of rural health needs should be assessment-based and should focus on health care needs, demands, and deficits.

C. Planning
1. Planning requires the design of interventions to meet the goal of increased self-care for the entire aggregate.
2. It is necessary to prioritize health problems for community action based on incidence, prevalence, and mortality.
3. The plan must be designed and managed using innovative methods to meet the nursing goals for the rural aggregate.

4. Interventions are planned to reduce the number of people at risk by developing needed resources that impact the greatest number of people.

D. Implementation
1. Interventions are based on prioritized goals and use of existing and developed services.
2. Interventions should increase the knowledge, skills, and motivation of the rural aggregate to engage in self-care.

E. Evaluation—Evaluation determines which activities and interventions have been successful or have made a significant contribution to the health status in terms of cost, benefits, and goal attainment.

F. Preventive nursing care
1. In rural settings, the community health nurse provides for optimal health through primary health care and health promotion.
2. Secondary prevention efforts involve referrals for service and focus on collaboration with clinicians and patients to decrease impairments caused by disease.
3. Tertiary prevention is applied to the rural aggregate through use of self-help groups and other methods to minimize disability.

X. **Rural Health Research**
A. Rural health research is sparse, and studies are infrequently repeated.
B. Rural research priorities should focus on development of rural nursing theory, refinement of rural nursing practice, health care policy, rural health care delivery systems, and nursing approaches using community-based interventions directed at the three levels of prevention.

TEACHING STRATEGIES

1. Obtain information from your state health department on hospitals, physicians, and nurses in rural areas. This information is usually available on a county-by-county basis. Have the class examine maps outlining where health care is available and where care is lacking.
2. Ask students from rural areas to share problems related to access. What is done about medical emergencies? Where do women go for prenatal care and delivery? How far is the nearest hospital? What is the background of local nurses and physicians?

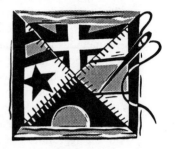

CHAPTER 17

Cultural Diversity and Community Health Nursing

ANNOTATED LEARNING OBJECTIVES

1. *Discuss racial and cultural diversity in U.S. society.*

    According to the United States Census, one third of the U.S. population consists of individuals from racial, ethnic, and cultural subgroups or minorities, and this is expected to increase to more than 50% within the next few decades.

    There are currently four federally defined minority groups in the United States: blacks, Hispanics, Asians, and Native Americans. Racial and cultural diversity create differences in the formation of values, family characteristics, socioeconomic status, education, religion, nutritional practices, and communication. Each of these differences may have an impact on health.

2. *Identify the cultural aspects of nursing care for culturally diverse individuals, groups, and communities.*

    Cultural beliefs and practices that influence nursing care of culturally diverse individuals, groups, and communities include values, norms, family characteristics, socioeconomic factors, education, occupation, family income, nutrition and dietary practices, and expressions of illness. Each of these should be assessed and the data included when planning care for minority and culturally diverse groups.

3. *Analyze the sociocultural, political, economic, and religious factors that impact the nursing care of culturally diverse individuals, groups, and communities.*

    Sociocultural factors that influence nursing care include family characteristics, values and norms, nutritional practices, developmental considerations, communication patterns, and health-related beliefs and practices.

Because of historical influences, socioeconomic status, and existing power structures, members of minority groups tend to have little political power. As a result, health care provision and access are often limited for these groups.

A disproportionate number of individuals from racially and ethnically diverse subgroups are members of the lower socioeconomic class, which influences their access to health care. Education is also linked to socioeconomic status; individuals in lower socioeconomic groups tend to be less educated.

Religion can affect health-related practices and health care by influencing values and attitudes about life and death. Prolongation of life, euthanasia, autopsy, donation of body for research, etc., are all influenced by religion. Related cultural practices, such as treatment of women by women in Muslim groups, influence how care is provided.

4. *Compare health-related values, beliefs, and practices of the dominant cultural group with those of individuals and groups from culturally diverse backgrounds.*

    The dominant cultural group in the United States is white, middle-class, and Protestant. This group typically believes in the fundamental goodness of human nature; demonstrates a desire to subdue, dominate, and control the environment; desires progress; maintains a futuristic orientation in which change is normal and progressive; is achievement-oriented; and stresses the importance of the individual.

    In contrast, other cultural groups may believe in the basic sinfulness of human nature; focus on being "one" with nature and allow nature to control events or allow a natural progression of events; maintain a past or present orientation that values tradition and ancestors; and stress the importance of the family or group over the individual.

5. *Apply the principles of transcultural nursing to community health nursing practice.*

When gathering data and applying the nursing process to transcultural nursing, the community health nurse should include a cultural assessment. The nurse should gather information about the ethnic origins of the cultural group, its values, and its methods of communication. The nurse should also become familiar with cultural sanctions and restrictions, health-related beliefs and practices, and nutritional issues within the culture. It is important to understand socioeconomic considerations and to know which organizations provide cultural support for the aggregate. The educational background and religious affiliation of the individuals can affect health care efforts, as can the cultural aspects of disease incidence, biocultural variations and developmental considerations. Additionally, community health nurses should become aware of their own cultural beliefs, values, and practices. The nurse should recognize political aspects of health care related to cultural issues and work to increase cultural sensitivity. Finally, when planning for care, the nurse should identify culturally-based health practices to incorporate or discourage in the plan of care.

LECTURE OUTLINE

I. **Transcultural Perspectives on Community Health Nursing**

   A. It is important for community health nurses to remember that all individuals, families, groups, communities, and institutions, including nurses and the nursing profession, have cultural characteristics that influence health.
   B. Culturally competent community health nursing requires that the nurse understand the lifestyle, value system, and health and illness behaviors of diverse individuals, families, groups, and communities, as well as the culture of institutions that influence the health and well-being of communities.

II. **Population Trends**
   A. By the year 2000, more than one quarter of the U.S. population will consist of individuals from the four federally defined minority groups.
      1. Blacks of African or Caribbean descent
      2. Hispanics
      3. Asians

      4. American and Alaskan natives
   B. It is predicted that by the early part of the twenty-first century, more than 50% of the population will be from culturally diverse backgrounds.
   C. Only about 9% of all nurses are from racial-ethnic minority backgrounds.
   D. Given the multicultural composition of the United States, nurses need to understand and meet the health needs of culturally diverse individuals, groups, and communities.

III. **Historical Perspective on Cultural Diversity**
   A. Florence Nightingale is credited as being concerned with cultural aspects of nursing care.
   B. In the early 1900s, public health nurses provided nursing care for European immigrants, often in tenement houses in New York City.
   C. In the 1960s and 1970s, nurses responded to the civil rights movement with increased sensitivity to individual attitudes, values, beliefs, and practices concerning health, illness, and caring among culturally diverse clients. In addition, the nursing profession responded with the development of a subspecialty of "transcultural nursing."

IV. **Transcultural Nursing in the Community**
   A. Definition and origin of transcultural nursing
      1. Transcultural nursing as a subspecialty was first identified in 1959 by Madeleine Leininger to describe the philosophical and theoretical similarities between nursing and anthropology.
      2. Leininger later wrote the first book on transcultural nursing, which she defined as "a formal area of study and practice focused on a comparative analysis of different cultures and subcultures in the world with respect to cultural care, health and illness beliefs, values, and practices, with the goal of using this knowledge to provide culture-specific and culture-universal nursing care to people."
      3. The term *cross-cultural nursing* is sometimes used synonymously with the term *transcultural nursing.*
      4. Leininger's theory is concerned with describing, explaining, and projecting nursing similarities and differences focused primarily on human care and caring in human cultures.
   B. Culture in transcultural nursing
      1. Culture refers to the complex whole, including knowledge, belief, art, morals, law,

customs, and any other capabilities and habits acquired by virtue of the fact that one is a member of a particular society.

2. Culture has four basic characteristics.
   a. It is learned from birth through the process of language acquisition and socialization.
   b. It is shared by all members of the same cultural group.
   c. It is adapted to specific conditions related to environmental and technical factors and to the availability of natural resources.
   d. It is dynamic.
3. A subculture is a large aggregate that shares characteristics that are not common to all members of the culture and that enable them to be a distinguishable subgroup.
   a. Within cultures, groups of individuals share beliefs, values, and attitudes that are different from those of other groups within the same culture.
   b. These differences are due to ethnicity, religion, education, occupation, age, and gender.
   c. Examples of U.S. subcultures based on ethnicity are blacks, Hispanics, Native Americans, and Chinese-Americans; subcultures based on religion include Catholics, Jews, Mormons, and Muslims.

C. Formation of values
1. *Value* refers to a desirable or undesirable state of affairs.
2. Values are a universal feature of all cultures, although the types and expression of values differ widely.
3. Norms are the rules by which human behavior is governed and are the result of the cultural values held by a group. Norms specify appropriate and inappropriate behavior.
4. All societies have a dominant value orientation that is shared by the majority of their members. This orientation is a result of early common experiences.
   a. In the United States, the dominant cultural group is composed of white, middle-class Protestants.
   b. In U.S. culture, this dominant value orientation includes belief in the fundamental goodness of human nature (although human nature may be viewed as a combination of good and evil); a desire to subdue, dominate, and control natural environment; belief in progress; a futuristic orientation in which change is viewed as normal and progressive; action and achievement orientation; and stressing the importance of the individual and the equality of all people.
   c. Values of this group include educational achievement, science, technology, individual expression, democracy, experimentation, and informality.

V. **Family**
A. In the United States, the family is the basic social unit.
B. There are three major categories of families.
   1. Nuclear (husband, wife, and children)
   2. Single parent (mother or father and children)
   3. Extended family (grandparents, aunts, uncles, cousins); minority families have traditionally been categorized as extended rather than nuclear families.
C. Family characteristics
   1. In addition to structural differences in families from different cultures, there may be functional diversity. Shared housing across families is an example. Families in non-dominant cultures (such as black and Hispanic families) tend to have larger numbers of both adults and children sharing residences.
   2. More than half of all black children under the age of three are born into single-parent families. Grandmothers play a dominant role in rearing their grandchildren in many black families.
   3. Both blacks and Hispanics have higher percentages of births to mothers under the age of 20 than do whites.
   4. When providing care for infants and children, it is important to identify the primary provider of care and to realize that this person may or may not be the biological parent.
   5. Families from ethnic minorities are often more conservative in roles and parenting practices than are white families. Traditional Japanese-American and Mexican-American families are family-centered, enforce strict sex and age roles, and emphasize children's respect for authority figures.

VI. **Socioeconomic Factors**
A. Socioeconomic status is a composite of the economic status of a family based on income,

wealth, occupation, educational attainment, and power.

1. Socioeconomic status is a measure of economic differences and the manner in which families live as a result of their economic well-being.
2. Most families with racially or ethnically diverse backgrounds have a lower socioeconomic status than does the population at large.

B. Distribution of resources

1. In the United States, a very small percentage of the population enjoys most of the nation's resources, primarily through ownership of corporations, real estate, and similar assets.
2. The U.S. population has traditionally been divided into three social classes: upper, middle, and lower. A disproportionate number of individuals from racially and ethnically diverse subgroups are members of the lower socioeconomic class, whereas a larger percentage of members of the dominant cultural group belong to the upper and middle classes.
3. In 1990, the median income of white families was about $37,000; in black families, it was $21,400; and in Hispanic families, it was $21,400.
4. Approximately 11% of white families fall below the poverty level, compared with 32% of black families and 38% of Hispanic families. This inequality of socioeconomic status has dramatically influenced the health care system.
5. The United States provides excellent health care to those with the highest socioeconomic status and poor health care to those with low socioeconomic status. Thus, the quality of health care is determined largely by one's socioeconomic status, not by health status.

C. Education is a component of socioeconomic status. Native Americans have the lowest education level of any major U.S. ethnic group.

VII. **Culture and Nutrition**—Food is an integral part of cultural identity.

A. Nutritional assessment of culturally diverse groups

1. Nutritional assessment should include cultural definition of food, form and content of ceremonial meals, amount and types of food eaten, and regularity of food consumption.

2. Social contacts and etiquette during meals also vary from culture to culture.

B. Although there are frequent differences in the dietary practices of cultural groups, aggregate dietary preferences among people from certain cultural groups can be described in terms of characteristic dishes and methods of food preparation.

C. Religion and diet

1. Cultural food preferences are often related to religious dietary beliefs and practices.
2. Many religions have proscriptive dietary practices and may use food as symbols in celebrations and rituals.
3. Knowing the client's religious practice as it relates to food makes it possible to suggest improvements or modifications that will not conflict with religious dietary laws.

VIII. **Culture and Religion**

A. Knowledge of health-related beliefs and practices, as well as general information about the religious observances, is important in providing culturally sensitive nursing care. Important holidays, days of religious worship, and important religious observances should be considered when scheduling care.

B. Religion and spirituality

1. Religious concerns evolve from and respond to the mysteries of life and death, good and evil, and pain and suffering. Nurses frequently encounter clients who find themselves searching for a spiritual meaning to help explain illness or disability.
2. Although very important, spiritual assessment may be very difficult for the nurse because of the abstract and personal nature of the topic.
3. Comfort with one's own spiritual beliefs is the foundation to effective assessment of spiritual needs in clients.
4. There is a distinction between religion and spirituality.
   a. Religion is an organized system of beliefs concerning the cause, nature, and purpose of the universe, especially belief in, and the worship of, a god or gods.
   b. Spirituality is composed of a person's unique life experience and personal effort to find purpose and meaning in life.
5. Prolongation of life, euthanasia, autopsy, donation of body for research, disposal of body and body parts (including fetus), and type of burial may be influenced by religious and spiritual beliefs. Discretion in

asking clients and their families about these issues is very important.

C. Developmental considerations
1. Childhood—Illness during childhood may present difficult clinical situations.
   a. Parental perceptions about the illness of their child may be influenced by religious beliefs.
   b. Parents may delay seeking medical care because they believe prayers should be tried first.
   c. Certain types of treatment (administration of blood or medications that contain caffeine or other prohibited substances) and selected procedures may be perceived as culturally taboo and may be prohibited by parents.
2. Old age
   a. Values such as independence, productivity, and self-reliance, which are held by the dominant U.S. culture, influence aging members of society.
   b. Americans define people at the chronological age of 65 as "old" and limit their work. In other cultures, people are identified as being unable to work, then are labeled as "old." The wisdom, not the productivity, of the elder is valued.
   c. Retirement is culturally defined. Some elderly people work as long as physical health continues; others continue to be active but assume less physically demanding jobs.
   d. In the dominant U.S. culture, a sense of integrity in accepting responsibility for their own lives is the main task of the elderly. In other cultures, such as Asian and Hispanic cultures, the elderly are often cared for by family members who welcome them into their homes when they are no longer able to live alone. Placement of an elderly family member in an institutional setting to be cared for by total strangers is seen as uncaring, impersonal, and culturally unacceptable by many groups.

IX. **Cross-Cultural Communication**
A. Both verbal and nonverbal communication are influenced by the cultural background of both the nurse and the client and are important in community health nursing.
B. *Cross-cultural communication* is the communication process that occurs between a nurse and a client who have different cultural backgrounds in which each attempts to understand the other's point of view from a cultural perspective.
1. Community health nurses are in a continuous process of communication. To ensure that a mutually respectful relationship is established, it is important for the nurse to introduce herself and indicate how the client is to address her (first name, last name, or title). The nurse should ask the client to do the same.
2. To care successfully for clients from other cultures, the nurse must overcome his or her own ethnocentrism. *Ethnocentrism* is the tendency to view one's own way of life as the most desirable, acceptable, or best, and to act as if one's culture is superior to another culture.
3. Cultural imposition, the tendency to impose one's own beliefs, values, and patterns of behavior on individuals from another culture, should be avoided.
C. Space, distance, and intimacy
1. Culturally appropriate distance zones vary widely.
2. Interactions between clients and nurses may depend on the client's desired degree of intimacy, which may range from very formal interactions to close personal relationships.
3. Clients of Hispanic, East Indian, or Middle Eastern origin may invade the nurse's personal space in an attempt to bring the nurse closer to them, and they may be puzzled by the nurse's movement away from them.
4. Some clients of Arab, Latin American, or Mediterranean origin may expect a high degree of intimacy and may attempt to involve the nurse in their family system by expecting participation in personal activities and social functions.
D. Overcoming communication barriers
1. Nurses tend to expect undemanding compliance, an attitude of respect for the care provider, and cooperation with requested behavior throughout the examination.
2. Individuals from diverse backgrounds may have different perceptions about the role of the individual and family in health care. During illness, culturally acceptable "sick role" behavior may range from aggressive, demanding behavior to silent passivity.
   a. Complaining, demanding behavior during illness is often rewarded with

attention among Jewish and Italian-American patients.
  b. Asian and Native American patients are likely to be quiet and compliant during illness.
  c. Asian clients may provide the nurse with the answers they think the nurse wants to hear; thus, the nurse should attempt to phrase questions or statements in a neutral manner that does not "lead" a response.
  E. Nonverbal communication
   1. It is very easy to overlook important information such as that conveyed by facial expressions, silence, eye contact, touch, or other body language.
   2. Communication patterns vary widely across cultures—even seemingly "innocent" behaviors such as smiling and handshaking.
   3. Sex issues may become significant; for example, men and women do not shake hands or touch each other in many Middle Eastern cultures.
   4. Interpretation of silence is important. People from some cultures find silence extremely uncomfortable, while others, such as Native Americans, consider silence essential to understanding and respecting the other person.
   5. Eye contact is among the most culturally variable nonverbal behaviors. Asian, native American, Indochinese, Arab, and Appalachian clients may consider direct eye contact impolite or aggressive, and they may avert their own eyes during the conversation.
  F. Touch
   1. In many cultures (Arab and Hispanic), male health care providers may be prohibited from touching or examining all or certain parts of the female body. The client may prefer female health care providers and may refuse to be examined by a man.
   2. Touching children may have special meaning in some cultures. Many Asians believe that strength resides in the head; therefore touching the head is considered disrespectful, and palpitation of fontanel of an infant of southeast Asian descent should be approached with sensitivity.
  G. Sex
   1. Violating norms related to male-female relationships among various cultures may jeopardize the nurse-client relationship. For

example, Arab-American women are never alone with a man (other than the husband).
   2. The best way to ensure that cultural variables have been considered is to ask the client about culturally relevant aspects of male-female relationships, preferably at the beginning of the interaction.
  H. Language
   1. Interviewing the non-English-speaking client requires a bilingual interpreter for full communication.
   2. Whenever possible, a bilingual team member or trained medical interpreter should be used. The interpreter is an important member of the health care team.
   3. There are two styles of interpreting.
    a. The line-by-line method ensures more accuracy, but takes more time.
    b. The summarizing method takes less time, but some information may inadvertently be lost.
   4. Simple language, not medical jargon, should always be used.

X. **Health-Related Beliefs and Practices**—The collection of data related to culturally based beliefs and practices regarding health and illness is very important. The nurse must understand the logic of the belief system underlying a given practice to understand the nature and meaning of the practice from the client's perspective.
  A. Health and culture
   1. It is important for the community health nurse to recognize that members of other cultures define "health" differently.
   2. Individuals may define themselves or others in their group as healthy even though the nurse identifies symptoms of disease.
  B. Defining illness from a cross-cultural perspective—Symptom labeling and diagnosis depend on the following factors.
   1. The degree of difference between the individual's behaviors and those the group has defined as normal
   2. The level of stigma attached to a particular set of symptoms
   3. Prevalence of pathology
   4. The meaning of the illness to the individual and family
  C. Causes of illness—There are three basic perspectives on disease causation: biomedical (scientific), naturalistic (holistic) and magico-religious. As a profession, nursing largely embraces the biomedical world view, although some aspects of holism have begun to gain

popularity. Belief in spiritual power is also held by many nurses who readily credit supernatural forces with various unexplained phenomena related to health and illness.

1. The biomedical theory of illness causation is based on the assumption that all events in life have a cause and an effect; that the human body functions more or less mechanically; that all life can be reduced or divided into smaller parts; and that all reality can be observed and measured. Most educational programs for nurses and other health care providers embrace biomedical theories to explain both physical and psychological illnesses.

2. The naturalistic (holistic) perspective is found most frequently among Native Americans, Asians, and others who believe that human life is only one aspect of nature and a part of the general order of the cosmos. The forces of nature must be kept in natural balance or harmony. Many Asians believe in the *yin-yang theory,* in which health exists when all aspects of the person are in perfect balance. The yin-yang theory is the basis for Eastern or Chinese medicine and is commonly embraced by Asian-Americans. The naturalistic perspective posits that the laws of nature create imbalances, chaos, and disease.

3. In the magicoreligious perspective, the basic premise is that the world is seen as an arena in which supernatural forces dominate. The fate of the world, and those in it, depends on the action of supernatural forces for good or evil. Examples of magical causes of illness include the belief in voodoo or witchcraft among some blacks and others from circum-Caribbean countries. Faith healing is based on religious beliefs and is most prevalent among certain Christian religions.

D. Culture and healing
1. In some cultures, the individual may turn to lay or folk-healing systems, religious healing, or biologic medicine. In addition to seeking help from the nurse as a biomedical health care provider, clients may also seek help from folk or religious healers.
2. Many clients (Hispanics or Native Americans) may believe that the cure is incomplete unless healing of mind, body, and spirit is accomplished. It is important for the nurse to be aware of alternative practices.

E. Folk healers
1. Each culture has its own healers, most of whom speak the native tongue of the client, make house calls, and cost significantly less than healers practicing in the biomedical system.
2. Hispanic clients may turn to a *curandero, espiritualista* (spiritualist), *yerbo* (herbalist), or *sabador* (chiropractor).
3. Black clients may mention having received assistance from a *hougan* (voodoo priest or priestess).
4. Native American clients may seek assistance from a *shaman* or medicine man.
5. Clients of Asian descent may visit herbalists, acupuncturists, or bone setters.
6. Many cultures have lay midwives or other health care providers who meet the needs of pregnant women.
7. Spiritual healers may be part of the ordained or official religious hierarchy.

XI. **Health, Illness, and Cultural Diversity**
A. Members of minority groups (blacks, Hispanics, Native Americans, and Asian/Pacific-Islanders) have not benefited equally in the U.S. health care system.
1. Although there have been improvements in health and longevity, statistical trends show a persistent disparity in health indicators among subgroups of the population.
2. Life expectancy is 4.5 years longer for whites than blacks, and the infant death rate for blacks is twice the rate for whites.
B. Causes of disease in minority populations
1. The term "excess deaths" is used to express the difference between the number of deaths actually observed in a minority group and the number of deaths that would have occurred in that group if it experienced the same death rates as the white population.
2. Rates of deaths from cancer, cardiovascular disease and stroke, chemical dependency (measured by deaths due to cirrhosis of the liver), diabetes, homicides and accidents, and infant mortality for minorities are higher than those for white populations.
3. Many causes of morbidity are higher for minority groups.

XII. **Cultural Expression of Illness**—There is wide cultural variation in the manner in which symptoms and disease conditions are perceived, diagnosed, labeled, and treated. Bodily symptoms are also perceived and reported in a variety of ways.

A. Cultural expression of pain
1. Pain is a universally recognized phenomenon; it is a private, subjective experience that is greatly influenced by cultural heritage.
2. Expectations, manifestations, and management of pain are all embedded in a cultural context.
3. The definition of pain is culturally determined, and nurses should expect variations in the expression of pain.
B. Culture-bound syndromes
1. Culture-bound syndromes are conditions that are culturally defined and may have no equal in another culture.
   a. Anorexia nervosa and bulimia are found almost exclusively in white Americans.
   b. *Empacho, mal ojo* and *susto* are found in Hispanic cultures.
2. More than 150 culture-bound syndromes have been documented by medical anthropologists.

XIII. Culture and treatment
A. After a symptom is identified, the first effort at treatment is often self-care. Self-care is preferred due to the inconvenience associated with traveling to a physician, nurse practitioner, or pharmacist; it is also less expensive.
B. Nontraditional interventions are gaining recognition by health care professionals in the biomedical health care system. The following interventions may be used alone or in combination with other treatments.
1. Acupuncture or acupressure
2. Therapeutic touch
3. Massage
4. Biofeedback
5. Relaxation techniques
6. Meditation
7. Hypnosis
8. Imagery
9. Herbal remedies

XIV. Cultural Negotiation
A. Cultural negotiation is an act of translation in which messages, instructions, and belief systems are manipulated, linked, or processed between the professional and the lay providers of treatment.
B. Cultural negotiation is used when conceptual differences exist between the client and the nurse.
C. In cultural negotiation, the nurse provides scientific information while acknowledging that the client may hold different views.

D. If the client's desired behaviors are helpful, positive, adaptive, or neutral, it is appropriate for the nurse to include these in the plan of care. If the behaviors are harmful, negative, or nonadaptive, the nurse should attempt to shift the client's perspective to that of the practitioner.

XV. Solutions to Health Care Problems in Culturally Diverse Populations—Health status is influenced by the interaction of physiological, cultural, psychological, and societal factors that are poorly understood for the general population and even less so for minorities. Diversity within and among minorities necessitates activities, programs and data collection that are tailored to meet the unique health care needs of many different subgroups.
A. Health information
1. Minority populations are less knowledgeable or aware of some health problems than are whites.
   a. Blacks and Hispanics receive less information about cancer and heart disease than do non-minority groups
   b. Blacks tend to underestimate the prevalence of cancer, ignore warning signs, and obtain fewer screening tests; they are generally diagnosed at later stages of cancer than are whites.
   c. Hispanic women receive less information about breast cancer than do white women.
   d. Many professionals and laypeople are not aware that heart disease is as common in black men as it is in white men.
   e. Mexican-Americans cultural attitudes regarding obesity and diet are often barriers to achieving weight control.
2. Many programs have been developed to address these and related concerns by promoting public awareness of these health problems.
B. Education
1. Planning health education programs requires sensitivity to cultural factors.
2. Meeting the language and cultural needs of each identified minority group, using minority-specific community resources to tailor educational approaches, and developing materials and methods of presentation that are commensurate with the educational level of the target population are essential considerations in the planning process.
3. Health programs should be sustained over a long period.

4. Education should be interpersonal.
5. The success of an education effort is often determined by the credibility of the source and depends on the skill and sensitivity of the nurse in communicating information in a culturally appropriate manner.
C. Delivery and financing of health services— Health care delivery models for minority populations should provide methods to achieve the following goals.
   1. Increase flexibility of health care delivery
   2. Facilitate access to services
   3. Improve efficiency of service and payment systems
   4. Modify services to be more culturally acceptable
D. Continuity of care
   1. Continuity of care is associated with improved health outcomes.
   2. Many of the major killers of minorities, such as cancer, heart disease and diabetes, are chronic rather than acute, requiring extended treatment regimens.
E. Financing problems
   1. Because of economic inequalities, members of minority groups tend to rely on Medicaid and charity for their health care needs.
      a. Proportionately, three times as many Native Americans, blacks, Hispanics, and some Asian groups as whites live in poverty.
      b. Proportionately, twice as many blacks and three times as many Hispanics as whites have no medical insurance.
      c. Of those without insurance, more than one third have not seen a physician during the last year.
   2. Elderly minority people are less likely to supplement Medicare with additional insurance.
F. Health professions development—Health professional organizations, academic institutions, state governments, health departments, and other groups should develop strategies to improve the availability and accessibility of health care to minority communities.
G. Developing strategies within the federal and nonfederal sectors
   1. Activities to improve health among minorities should involve organizations at all levels—community, municipal, state, and national.
   2. Community involvement in developing health promotion activities can contribute

to their success by providing credibility and visibility to the activities and facilitating their acceptance.
H. Improving and using available sources of data
   1. Inclusion of racial and ethnic identifiers in databases and oversampling of selected minorities in national surveys should improve existing sources of health data.
   2. Data set analysis is needed to assist in understanding the health status and needs of minority populations.

XVI. **Role of the Community Health Nurse in Improving Health for Culturally Diverse People—** Research studies suggest that community health nurses do not feel confident in caring for any of the major ethnic groups. The following principles may assist the community health nurse when working with culturally diverse clients.
A. Cultural assessment—The cultural assessment is used to determine and appraise traits and characteristics of the culture to which the client belongs. This is as vital as a physical and psychological assessment and should include the following elements.
   1. A brief history of the ethnic and racial origins of the cultural group with which the client identifies
   2. Values orientation (attitudes, values and beliefs about health, birth, death, illness, etc.)
   3. Cultural sanctions and restrictions
   4. Communication (language spoken; nonverbal communication patterns)
   5. Health-related beliefs and practices (restrictions, actions, and expectations)
   6. Nutrition
   7. Socioeconomic considerations
   8. Organizations providing cultural support
   9. Educational background
   10. Religious affiliation
   11. Cultural aspects of disease incidence
   12. Biocultural variations (physical or anatomical features characteristic of that racial or ethnic group)
   13. Developmental considerations (roles and expectations of children, women, and the elderly)
B. Cultural self-assessment—Identification of health-related attitudes, values, beliefs, and practices that are part of the nurse's culture allows better understanding of the cultural aspects of health care.
C. Knowledge about local cultures—Community health nurses should learn about the culturally

diverse characteristics of the most prevalent subgroups within the community.
D. Recognition of political aspects—Awareness of political aspects of health care can enable the nurse to have increased involvement in influencing legislation and funding priorities aimed at improving health care for specific populations.
E. Provision of culturally competent care —The community health nurse applies the nursing process in a manner that is culturally sensitive, relevant and appropriate. The nurse should be aware of cultural similarities and differences between the nurse and the client.
F. Recognition of culturally based health practices
   1. Once health practices are understood, a determination regarding their appropriateness in a particular context can be made.
   2. Helpful and neutral practices should be encouraged or "tolerated," whereas harmful practices should be discouraged.
G. Federal resources
   1. U.S. Department of Health and Human Services (DHHS)—Federal resources are available for improving health care of federally defined minority populations through the DHHS. Agencies include the U.S. Public Health Service, the Office of Minority Health and Indian Health Services.
   2. Office of Minority Health—The Office of Minority Health coordinates federal efforts to improve the health status of racial and ethnic minority populations. The OMH was created to establish short- and long-range goals and objectives and to coordinate DHHS activities to achieve the following aims, among others.
      a. Prevent disease, promote health, deliver service, and perform research on minority health
      b. Create a national minority health resource center
      c. Support research, demonstrations and evaluations of new and innovative models to increase understanding of risk factors
      d. Support information dissemination and health education efforts in minority communities in addition to other duties.
H. Initiatives for improved minority health care—"Program Direction 9: Improving the Health of Minority and Low-Income People" is a plan to address the health and social service efforts of the DHHS to improve the health of these

groups. This program is designed to reduce disparities in premature death, chronic disease, and injuries by improving access to health care and reducing risks of chronic disease and conditions that disproportionately affect minority and low-income people.
   I. Grant programs—The Office of Minority Health has grants to help communities deal with specific problems. Examples include the Minority Community Health Coalition Demonstration Grant Program and the Minority Human Immunodeficiency Virus Education and Prevention Grant Program.
   J. Indian Health Service—The Indian Health Service is the agency within the Public Health Service that is responsible for providing federal health services to American Indians and Alaskan natives. These services are based on constitutionally defined responsibilities and are designed to improve the health of these aggregates to the highest level possible.

XVII. **Research Agenda**—Research should be developed to investigate factors affecting minority health. Risk factor identification, risk factor prevalence, health education interventions, preventive interventions, treatments, and health outcomes should be examined closely.
A. Research on culture and community health nursing—Many resources are available for Community Health Nurses desiring information on the latest research regarding cultural aspects of community health nursing. Electronic bulletin boards, nursing journals and the Transcultural Nursing Society are examples.
B. Community health nursing and culturally diverse populations—Research has indicated that nurses are not being provided with experiences they need to build confidence in the application of community health concepts to the care of culturally diverse populations.

TEACHING STRATEGIES

1. Encourage students from racial or ethnic minorities to share differences in values, norms, religions and health beliefs. Have them discuss how these factors influence health practices and might impact health care delivery. Explore how students and nurses can develop sensitivity to others' beliefs.
2. Invite a health care provider who works with smaller minority groups such as refugees to speak to the class. Have the person provide specific examples of difficulties in planning and providing care for these aggregates.

3. Invite a speaker from the Public Health Service, Indian Health Service, or Office of Minority Health to speak to the class regarding health initiatives and research currently underway to improve the health of minority groups.

4. Review the *Healthy People 2000* objectives that relate to minority health. In small groups, have students discuss interventions to address the objectives. Ask each group to draft a community care plan related to one or more objectives.

CHAPTER

18

The African-American Community

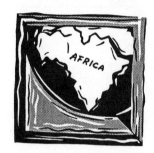

ANNOTATED LEARNING OBJECTIVES

1. *Identify the impact of social, economic, and cultural trends in U.S. society on the health of African-Americans.*

   Currently, African-Americans make up 12% of the U.S. population, and this is anticipated to grow to 15% by the year 2000. Average black family income is about half that of whites, with a much larger percentage of blacks living below the poverty level. Education levels are somewhat lower for African-Americans, and the number of single women as "head of household" is much larger. Blacks are more likely to be divorced and have children out of wedlock. Racism significantly influences the lives of African-Americans.

   Each of these facts serves to influence the health of African-Americans by lowering the level of health care they receive due to lack of access, inhibited ability to pay for health care, and less understanding of health promotion and prevention measures. As a result, "excess" death rates (rates greater than those of whites) are evident in at least six areas: cancer, infant mortality, cardiovascular disease, homicide, cirrhosis, and unintentional injuries.

2. *Assess the community health nursing needs of African-American individuals, families, and communities.*

   Community health nursing interventions for African-Americans should be directed toward the excess causes of morbidity and mortality found in this population. Efforts to reduce cancer and cardiovascular deaths should include education on prevention, as well as early detection and treatment.

Efforts to reduce dependency on alcoholism and the use of illegal drugs should focus on education. Community efforts should focus on the improvement of social and economic opportunities for African-Americans.

Infant mortality may be reduced through pregnancy prevention and increasing accessibility to comprehensive prenatal care. Finally, reduction of deaths from homicide may be accomplished through legal and cultural efforts to reduce family violence, childhood aggression, alcoholism, and drug abuse.

3. *List the cultural precepts that characterize African-American world view.*

   In the traditional African-American community, the world view has been guided by eight cultural precepts that reflect ancient African metaphysics. The cultural precepts are:
   - Consubstantiation—All things have the same essence (force and spirit).
   - Interdependence—All things are interconnected and interrelated.
   - Egalitarianism—All things are the same and equal and in harmonious interaction.
   - Collectivism—The individual is part of a larger whole whose survival is dependent on the collective survival.
   - Transformation—All things are striving to function at a higher and greater level.
   - Cooperation—Cooperation is necessary for the transformation and survival of the group.
   - Humaneness—Humaneness guides the individual's relationship and behavior with others and ensures mutual cooperation, collectivism, egalitarianism, cohesiveness, and collective survival.

- Synergism—The collective effort is greater than the individual effort in bringing about transformation and change.

4. Identify ways in which community health nurses can provide culturally sensitive and culturally competent care for African-American individuals, families, and communities.

To increase cultural sensitivity, community health nurses can first seek to understand historical and social factors that have influenced the evolution of the African American culture. Nurses should identify their own cultural attitudes and beliefs about African-Americans by performing a cultural self-assessment. Nurses should be aware of cultural stereotypes and biocultural physical variations in African-Americans and should be culturally sensitive in their recommendations and suggestions.

5. Analyze the major causes of excess morbidity and mortality among African-Americans and their sociopolitical causes.

Excess morbidity and mortality among African-Americans can be traced to several factors. Cancer deaths are higher for African-Americans due to delay in detection, lower socioeconomic status, and treatment differences due to cultural or financial factors, biological factors, nutrition, and diet.

Excess morbidity and mortality from cardiovascular causes can be linked to higher incidences of hypertension and smoking in black men. In black women, cardiovascular causes include higher incidences of diabetes and obesity.

Homicide is the leading cause of death for young black men. Homicide levels are attributed to psychosocial problems, poor economic environment, lifestyles, and substance use.

Infant mortality rates for blacks are about twice that for whites. This may be due to poor socioeconomic status, educational levels, high teenage pregnancy rates, poor nutrition, substance abuse, or lack of prenatal care.

6. Propose solutions to the community health problems facing African-American individuals, families, and groups.

Primary, secondary, and tertiary prevention efforts should be instituted with an awareness of cultural beliefs and health practices. Efforts to reduce "excess deaths" should include interventions such as health education for prevention and early detection of cancer; improved access to affordable, comprehensive health care, particularly for pregnant women and small children; encouragement of contraception use to prevent unwanted pregnancies;

and early detection and control of hypertension and diabetes.

7. List the six profiles of African-Americans.

African-American identity typically aligns along one of six dimension or profiles. These are:

- Acculturated—resemble Euro-Americans in thought, behavior, and beliefs. Human and personal needs are met within the Euro-American environment.
- Bicultural—can move between the African-American and white cultures. They adopt roles and behaviors similar to the group with which they are interacting. Survival needs are met predominately within the white culture, but personal needs are met within the African-American community.
- Culturally immersed conformist—have a strong sense of racial pride and identity. Their survival needs are met within the white community, but their interaction with whites is limited to the work environment.
- Culturally immersed Afrocentric—have a strong self-identity as African-American. They desire to build a powerful and economically independent black community.
- Culturally immersed deviant—are generally distrustful of whites and acculturated and bicultural African-Americans. Value systems are opposite those of whites, and most of their personal and survival needs are met in the African-American community.
- Traditional unacculturated—are usually older and have strong spiritual values. Their survival needs are met in the white community, and their human needs are met in the African-American community. They see integration as necessary but do not value assimilation. They support a "color-blind society."

LECTURE OUTLINE

I. **African-American History**
   A. Remnants of Ancient-African thought, cultural traditions, and values have contributed to contemporary identity.
   B. Historically, Africans first came to North America in 1619 (one year before the Pilgrims).
      1. The earliest African settlers were not slaves but free men and women working as indentured servants.
      2. Between 1619 and 1860, more than 4 million Africans were brought to North America, primarily from the west coast of Africa.

3. Since that time, Africans and their descendants have come to the United States from other parts of Africa as well as from many Caribbean nations.
4. The Civil War (1860s) freed black slaves.
C. During the 20th century, African-Americans have continually sought to win equal civil rights. Serious inequality still exists in many areas, including health care.

II. African-Americans in Contemporary Society
A. Sociodemographic overview
1. According to the Bureau of the Census, African-Americans constitute 12.1% of the U.S. population (1990) and by the year 2000, this will climb to 15%.
2. Thirty-three percent of African-Americans are younger than 18.
3. Males are over-represented in the 18-year-old and younger group.
4. Older women are disproportionately represented in the 65-year-old and older group.
B. Rural vs. urban African-Americans —The majority of African-Americans live in metropolitan or urban areas, but significant numbers also reside in rural parts of the country, particularly in the South.
C. Socioeconomic apartheid: poverty
1. Black family income is only 56% of white family income.
2. Black family incomes must be used to support more family members, and both husband and wife are employed in more black families than in white families.
3. The majority of female-headed black families live below the poverty level.
4. More than one third of the U.S. black population lives in poverty, compared with 12% of the white population. Children are disproportionally affected.
5. Twenty-five percent of poor blacks receive public assistance.
6. Unemployment for blacks is higher than for whites, particularly for black teenagers.
D. Education
1. Approximately 66% of African-Americans have completed high school, compared with almost 80% of whites.
2. African-American women tend to have more education than African-American men.
3. College-educated whites face fewer barriers to career aspirations than do college-educated African-Americans.

III. Social Justice: An African-American Perspective
A. Self-concept, racism, and racial identity
1. Racial identity and self-concept are interrelated.
   a. African-Americans share a distinct and unique immigrant history which is different from other immigrant groups in that they were forcibly transplanted from Africa; endured chattel slavery; and continue to endure a hostile and oppressive environment.
   b. Virtually every African-American knows despair, humiliation, and loss of dignity as a consequence of skin color.
   c. Hostile behaviors may range from anger hidden by smiles to overt acting out of aggression with violence.
2. African-American identity reflects a process of socialization and contact with an oppressive and violent society. As a result of socialization, African-Americans develop a functional sense of inferiority. This process of racism operates within the family, the community, and society.
B. Profiles of African-Americans—African-American identity typically aligns along one of six dimension or profiles.
1. Acculturated
   a. Resemble Euro-Americans in thought, behavior, and beliefs
   b. Human and personal needs are met within the Euro-American environment
2. Bicultural
   a. Move between the African-American and white cultures
   b. Adopt roles and behaviors similar to the group with which they are interacting at a given time
   c. Survival needs are met predominately within the white culture, but their personal needs are met within the African-American community
3. Culturally immersed conformist
   a. Have a strong sense of racial pride and identity
   b. Survival needs are met within the white community, but interaction with whites is limited to the work environment
4. Culturally immersed Afrocentric
   a. Have a strong self-identity as African-American
   b. Desire to build a powerful and economically independent black community

5. Culturally immersed deviant
   a. Generally distrustful of whites and of acculturated and bicultural African-Americans
   b. Value systems are opposite of those of whites
   c. Most of personal and survival needs are met within the African-American community
6. Traditional unacculturated
   a. Usually older
   b. Have strong spiritual values
   c. Survival needs are met in the white community, and human needs are met in the African-American community
   d. See integration as necessary, but do not value assimilation
   e. Support a "color-blind society"
C. Racism
   1. Racism can be redefined as a form of violence characterized by one group's persistent and continuous efforts to dominate and control another.
   2. Organizational, institutional, and individual racism constitutes one of the major stressors in the lives of African-Americans.
   3. Racism reinforces African-Americans' position of social marginality and contributes to persistent disparities in important indicators of living conditions such as health, morbidity, and mortality.
D. African-American cultural beliefs
   1. Cultural beliefs guide African-American behavior.
   2. Contemporary behavior, values and beliefs of African-Americans reflect a dynamic interplay between the political, social, and economic realities affecting their lives.
E. African-American world view and cultural precepts
   1. In the traditional African-American community, the world view has been guided by eight cultural precepts that reflect ancient African metaphysics.
      a. Consubstantiation—All things have the same essence (force and spirit).
      b. Interdependence—All things are interconnected and interrelated.
      c. Egalitarianism—All things are the same and equal and in harmonious interaction.
      d. Collectivism—The individual is part of a larger whole whose survival is dependent on the collective survival.
      e. Transformation—All things are striving to function at a higher and greater level.
      f. Cooperation—Cooperation is necessary for the transformation and survival of the group.
      g. Humaneness—Humaneness guides the individual's relationship and behavior with others, ensuring cooperation, collectivism, egalitarianism, cohesiveness. and collective survival.
      h. Synergism—Synergism is a cooperative, collective effort that is greater than the sum of the individual efforts in bringing about transformation and change.
   2. Spiritually gives African-Americans a transcendent meaning of life.
      a. Religion and spiritually provide the aggregate with a framework to understand struggle.
      b. God is the creator of all, and all things are endowed with force and spirit.
      c. All cultural precepts are evident in the spiritual practices of African-Americans.
F. Changing patterns of African-American family life
   1. African-American families typically consist of an extended network.
   2. Members of the "family" may not necessarily be related by birth or marriage.
   3. The family often has strong kinship ties and shares family roles.
   4. Roles are determined by ability rather than by gender or marital association.
   5. Children are considered vitally important.
G. Gender roles
   1. African-American men have often been deprived of economic opportunity to perform normal masculine functions of providing for their families.
   2. Unemployment rates, increased use of drugs and alcohol, high suicide rate, declining life expectancy, increased crime rate, and poor performance in school all serve to alter traditional sex roles for African-American males.
   3. The African-American dyad is characterized by more equal roles and economic parity. African-American women have never traditionally been dependent on the males.
   4. Lower-class African-American women tend to be the breadwinners, enjoy higher levels of education than their male coun-

terparts, and hold dominant positions in their families.
5. There are more African-American females than males.
6. African-American wives are usually less satisfied with their marriages than are white wives.

IV. **Communication and Language**
   A. Black English has been referred to as black dialect, black Creole, soul talk, Afro-American speech, ebonics, and Afro.
      1. It is a dialect spoken at some time by 80-90% of African-Americans.
      2. Black English is essentially Euro-American speech with African-American meaning, nuance, tone, and gesture.
   B. Development of black English
      1. During slavery, West African slaves developed pidgin to communicate among themselves as well as with whites. *Pidgin* is a form of communication used when two persons speak two different languages and do not have a common third language.
      2. Offspring of the early slaves began to speak English pidgin, which developed into Creole. In Creole, West African structure and idiom are retained, but English words are substituted.
   C. Characteristics of black English
      1. Black English is highly oral, stylized, rhythmic, and spontaneous rather than an exact, precise language.
      2. The meanings of words are conveyed by the manner in which they are said (intonation and inflection).
      3. Linguistic aspects of Black English include grammatical structure and word usage.
      4. When working with members of this aggregate, community health nurses should use characteristics of African-American communication, such as incorporating oral and visual approaches, when teaching about issues related to health.

V. **Health Beliefs and Practices**
   A. Traditional beliefs about health and illness
      1. In African-American culture, a healthy person is in harmony with nature; illness occurs with disharmony.
      2. Traditional beliefs about health are holistic, with mind, body, and spirit being integrally interwoven.
      3. Illness is a product of interaction with the environment or a product of disharmony with the environment.

4. Illness may be either natural or unnatural.
   a. Natural illnesses are linked to inappropriate self-care (exposure to toxins, pollutants, cold).
   b. Unnatural illnesses are the result of forces (witchcraft, voodoo, or punishment for transgressions against others).
5. The goal of treatment from the traditional African perspective is to remove the harmful spirit(s) from the body of the ill person.
   B. Sociopolitical variations in health and illness
      1. The health status of African-Americans is a function of historic and contemporary forces, economics, and power imbalances.
      2. There is a disparity in the health status of African-Americans compared with Euro-Americans.
         a. Life expectancy for African-Americans is 69.8 years, compared with 76.5 years for Euro-Americans.
         b. Life expectancy is 73.9 years for African-American women and 65.5 years for African-American men.
      3. African-Americans have a higher death ratio than whites for HIV/AIDS (3.4:1), homicide and legal intervention (6.8:1), and perinatal conditions (2.1:1) when compared with whites.
      4. African-American have a disproportionately high incidence of hypertensive disease, diabetes, cancer, and glaucoma.
   C. Indicators of health in the African-American population
      1. Researchers attribute differences in mortality to poverty, poor housing conditions, chronic psychological stress, substance abuse, and inadequate access to medical care.
      2. Regardless of income, African-American men and women have higher rates of mortality than whites.
      3. African-Americans are dying earlier in life from preventable and treatable causes.
      4. Excess deaths among African-Americans between the ages of 45 and 69 years were mainly the result of cancer, heart disease, stroke, diabetes, and cirrhosis.
         a. Cardiovascular disease
            1) African-American men are almost twice as likely to die from stroke as are white men.
            2) For African-Americans ages 20-64 there is an excess mortality from coronary heart disease. This is more

marked in African-American women than in men. Related factors include hypertension (much more common among African-Americans, especially men); elevated cholesterol levels; smoking; and obesity.

  b. Infant mortality

    1) African-American females continue to have a higher ratio of infant mortality (2.1:1) in comparison to white women. Reasons include socioeconomic variables such as educational attainment, family stability and employment status; increased risk of delivering a low-birthweight infant (5.7% of white infants, compared with 13.5% of African American infants); increased risk of neonatal death among infants of normal birthweight; and increased risk of post-neonatal death.

    2) Risk factors associated with poor perinatal outcome among African-Americans include low income and inadequate insurance, preexisting disease conditions, poor nutrition, inadequate housing, limited maternal education, stressful work environment, disrupted families; lack of social support, and problems related to transportation and child care.

    3) Higher percentage of teen pregnancy and out-of-wedlock births contribute greatly to poor pregnancy outcomes.

  c. AIDS and HIV—AIDS is the eighth leading cause of death in the United States.

    1) The rates have risen in the intravenous drug user group, which affects a large number of African-Americans.

    2) African-American men have the highest age-adjusted death rate from AIDS.

    3) In 1991, 32% of all new cases of HIV infection were African-Americans.

    4) More than 72% of women with AIDS are non-white and 55% are African-American.

    5) African-American children account for more than half of all pediatric AIDS cases.

D. Alcohol problems—Alcohol abuse has a major impact on the health of African-Americans.

  1. African-American drinking patterns are similar to those for the general population, with rates varying greatly by geographical location, gender, and religion.

  2. A higher percentage of both abstainers and heavy drinkers are found in the female African-American community than in female whites.

  3. African-Americans experience substance-related health problems to a greater extent than whites. This is particularly manifested in higher arrests, homicides, unintentional injuries, and accidents.

  4. Men of both groups have similar patterns, although African-American men develop heavy drinking patterns later in life.

  5. Esophageal cancer rates and fetal alcohol syndrome are much higher for blacks.

E. Drug-related problems

  1. Inner-city African-Americans are at greater risk for drug abuse and its consequences.

    a. They have higher rates of marijuana, cocaine, heroine, and illicit methadone use than do whites.

    b. African-Americans are more likely than whites to be involved with more dangerous drugs, and to use more dangerous combinations of drugs.

  2. Risk factors for drug and alcohol related problems in African-American communities include the following.

    a. History of racism
    b. Poverty
    c. Unemployment
    d. Failure to eradicate drug trafficking in African-American communities
    e. The allure of, and rewards for, selling drugs
    f. Powerlessness
    g. Cultural and economic conditions that favor hustling and devalue menial jobs
    h. Peer pressure
    i. Frustration from confronting racism and discrimination
    j. High levels of stress

F. Homicide and unintentional injuries

  1. Although African-Americans comprise only 12% of the total population, they account for 43% of the homicide victims.

  2. Homicide is the leading cause of death for African-American males aged 15–44.

  3. Homicides rates are particularly high in the largest cities.

4. All of the following psychological factors contribute to increased homicide rates.
    a. Mental processes
    b. Physical, historical, cultural, social, educational, and economic environments
    c. Lifestyle
    d. Factors related to age and gender

VI. **Nursing Care of African-Americans**
  A. Serving the aggregate need
    1. Nurses working with African-Americans must be familiar with the problems and barriers that contribute to the health status of this population.
    2. Issues, strategies, and culturally relevant and sensitive nursing care should be designed and initated to address problems such as infant mortality, homicide, and AIDS/HIV prevention.
  B. Infant mortality
    1. *Primary prevention* should focus on avoidance of unwanted pregnancy and should target unprotected sexual activity.
    2. *Secondary prevention* efforts should target adolescent females who are pregnant.
      a. Efforts should address prevention of additional unintended pregnancies, appropriate sexual behavior, and the role of parents in the lives of their offspring.
      b. Early prenatal care must be encouraged.
  C. Homicide
    1. *Primary prevention* efforts should be directed at correcting the social, cultural, and legal aspects of the environment that facilitate perpetuation of the high homicide rates among African-Americans.
    2. *Secondary prevention* efforts should be directed toward individuals that manifest early signs of behavioral and social problems related to increased risk for homicide. Family violence, childhood aggression, school violence, alcoholism and drug abuse are important focal points for efforts aimed at secondary prevention.
    3. *Tertiary prevention* strategies to address homicide include efforts to reduce domestic violence, reduce the use of alcohol and drugs, and control gangs.
  D. AIDS and HIV prevention
    1. AIDS prevention should be culturally sensitive and multifactorial in nature.
    2. Prevention strategies should stress individual and collective group survival and transformation.

3. AIDS interventions should focus on the following strategies.
    a. Increasing perceived risk and perceived self-efficacy
    b. Altering negative outcome expectancies
4. Interventions should target knowledge of AIDS and should include a skills-building component to enhance self-efficacy.
5. Interventions should involve important members of the individual's support network.

VII. **Cultural Sensitivity**
  A. Culturally sensitive health care efforts
    1. Nurses who work with African-American groups or communities should strive to make care culturally sensitive.
    2. They should seek input from African-American nurses or other health care team members.
    3. When possible, key African-American community-based leaders should be part of planning, implementation, and evaluation of projects or programs to provide culturally sensitive health care.
  B. Cultural self-assessment
    1. Nurses caring for African-Americans should identify individual culturally-based attitudes and beliefs about African-Americans, race, prejudice, racial discrimination, and related issues.
    2. Self-assessment requires honesty and sincerity and necessitates reflection on parents, other family members, and close friends in terms of their attitude toward African-Americans.
  C. Cultural stereotypes
    1. A nurse should examine the cultural stereotype of African-Americans held by other members of the nurse's culture.
    2. The nurse should also examine the recent interactions between the two cultures in the local community.
  D. Roles of the community health nurse
    1. The roles of the community health nurse usually include advocate, educator, social policy analyst, outreach worker, and participant observer.
    2. When working with African-Americans, a nurse's prevention efforts should capitalize on cultural strengths within the community to facilitate functional competence and positive self-identity.
    3. Prevention efforts should seek to modify those environmental and societal factors

that continue to threaten the integrity of the aggregate.

3. Factors that hinder prevention efforts with African-American clients and community include internal resistance, cultural dissonance, Eurocentrism, and racial-cultural paranoia.

4. It is imperative that the community health nurse evaluate barriers that might undermine prevention efforts.

TEACHING STRATEGIES

1. Invite an African-American nurse to speak to the class about provision of health care to African-Americans. Encourage the speaker to discuss various aspects of racial differences that influence health and health care.

2. Have individual students complete cultural self-assessments and share their findings. Ask African-Americans to lead a discussion about perceived and actual differences between whites and blacks.

The Mexican-American Community

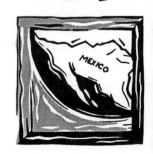

ANNOTATED LEARNING OBJECTIVES

1. *Identify the disease and health conditions prevalent among Mexican-Americans.*

   Mexican-Americans have higher rates of obesity and diabetes than white Americans. However, they have lower rates of cardiovascular disease. Although they have less prenatal care than the population at large, Mexican-Americans do not have a significantly higher number of low-birthweight infants. Mexican-American children with sight and hearing difficulties are less likely to be screened.

2. *Describe two major reasons for the lower health status of a large segment of the Mexican-American community.*

   Adverse socioeconomic conditions, including poverty and lack of education, contribute to the poorer health status of Mexican-Americans. Poverty can result in little money for medical services, particularly for preventive care. Lack of formal education results in lowered awareness of modern health care and less emphasis on health promotion. Crowded housing and lack of basic services result in a greater potential for spreading communicable diseases.

3. *Discuss factors that impede the Mexican-American from receiving health care.*

   Poverty, lack of education, language barriers and other communication problems, lack of transportation, and lack of telephones contribute to poor Mexican-American health by reducing access to health care. Provider hours are often difficult to keep because they coincide with working hours.

4. *Describe the folk health system that is unique to Mexican-Americans.*

   Mexican-Americans typically view health and disease as an area in which God and other spiritual forces are influential, either directly or indirectly. A particular illness may be a punishment from God or the result of a malevolent source of illness.

   Folk healing is very important in Mexican-American culture. The *curandero*, or healer, is a diagnostician, counselor, and practitioner who has derived powers of healing from God. Diseases are caused by empirical, magical, and psychological sources and may be the result of "hot/cold" imbalances. Herbal remedies, sometimes in conjunction with prayer, are used to treat various ailments.

5. *Apply knowledge of Mexican-American health and culture in planning culturally sensitive nursing care at the individual, family, and community levels.*

   The community health nurse should work within the available system to increase access to culturally sensitive health care for Mexican-Americans. Inclusion of the family in health care; home care, when possible; communication between the practitioner and patients; and use of bilingual and bicultural health practitioners should be encouraged. Health care should be within the Mexican-American social frame of reference, focusing on problems known to exist in the community. Community involvement, outreach, and comprehensive programs including health promotion and illness prevention should be advocated.

LECTURE OUTLINE

I. **Understanding Mexican-American Health Needs**

   A. Hispanics are the fastest-growing minority group in the United States. Typically, Hispanics are classified into five subgroups.

   1. Mexican-Americans

2. Puerto Ricans
3. Cuban-Americans
4. Central or South Americans
5. "Other" Hispanics
B. Compared with whites, Hispanics are more likely to live in poverty, be unemployed or under-employed, have little education, and have no private insurance.
C. Hispanics are at increased risk for certain medical conditions, including diabetes, hypertension, tuberculosis, acquired immunodeficiency syndrome, alcoholism, cirrhosis, some cancers, and violent death.
D. Beliefs and associated reactions to disease and illness fall into three broad categories.
   1. *Scientific reaction* is characterized by a logical explanation of events in relation to a cause and effect.
   2. *Nonscientific reaction* stems from the ancient belief that illness may be caused by magic or a supernatural source.
   3. *Folk medicine* is practiced throughout the world and has some basis in the scientific realm. Within the Mexican-American community, the folk medicinal practice is referred to as *curanderismo.*
E. Post-acculturation stress syndrome (PASS) predominately affects minority populations that have attempted to assimilate and become acculturated into the general and dominant population.
   1. The primary cause of PASS is the inability to assimilate into the dominant societal group effectively and completely.
   2. Contributing factors
      a. Mistrust of the dominant system
      b. Lack of opportunities to succeed in society
      c. Prejudice
      d. Lack of guidance for effective acculturation
      e. Culture shock
      f. Poverty
   3. Symptoms of PASS
      a. Lack of self-esteem
      b. Apathy
      c. Violence
      d. On-the-job injuries
      e. Alcoholism
      f. Gang involvement
   4. Interventions to prevent or minimize PASS
      a. Improve the educational status of Mexican-Americans
      b. Provide acculturation guidance

c. Provide support from the dominant culture
d. Increase the number of Mexican-American role models
e. Provide bilingual education in public schools
f. Provide counseling
g. Provide diversity training in business and industry
h. Improve correctional systems
i. Provide professional counseling
j. Provide professional rehabilitation

II. **Disease Prevalence in the Mexican-American Community and Access to Health Care**
   A. Level of health among Mexican-Americans
      1. Mexican-Americans have a lower socioeconomic status, higher rates of obesity and diabetes, and lower rates of cardiovascular disease than non-Hispanic whites.
      2. Many Mexican-Americans do not have a regular source of health care.
      3. Lower socioeconomic status may be both a cause and a result of Mexican-American health conditions.
      4. Almost one third of Mexican-Americans are without a regular source of health care.
   B. Disease prevalence
      1. Among the findings of HHANES (a national effort to measure the health of Mexican-Americans) was that routine vision, hearing, and dental examinations are not practiced among Mexican-American children.
      2. Prevalence of non-insulin-dependent diabetes was 2.5 times higher among Mexican-Americans than among non-Hispanic white Americans.
      3. Despite their lower socioeconomic status and higher rates of obesity and diabetes, Mexican-Americans have lower cardiovascular disease rates than whites.
   C. Effect of health on Mexican-American socioeconomic condition
      1. The most significant and consistent predictor of health status of Mexican-Americans is employment.
      2. Less acculturated men have poorer health.
      3. Poor health affects a person's socioeconomic condition adversely.
         a. Causes an interruption in or termination of employment
         b. Prevents an individual from learning new skills or participating in activities that would help increase income and education

c. Causes an individual to spend a disproportionate amount of income on maintaining health status

D. Effects of adverse socioeconomic conditions on health
1. Poor working conditions and benefits may affect health adversely in any of the following ways.
   a. Subject a person to unhealthy environmental conditions (housing, work, etc.)
   b. Deprive a person of the education necessary to understand preventive measures in disease control and general physical well-being
   c. Limit care received
   d. Bar a person from health care services
   e. Lead a person to seek types of health care that might be harmful
2. The relationship between poverty and health creates many problems.
   a. Low income results in little money for medical services; thus, people may be forced to forego medical services or rely on assistance from others (family, friends, charities, or public funds).
   b. Lack of formal education results in lowered awareness of modern preventive health care.
   c. Crowded housing and lack of basic services such as treated water and proper sewage disposal result in a greater potential for the spread of communicable diseases

III. **The Mexican-American Family**
A. By the year 2000, Hispanics will become the majority minority population.
1. The number of Hispanics in the United States (currently 20 million) will increase to 32 million by the year 2010.
2. One third to one half of the 6–10 million Mexican-Americans currently live near or below the official level of poverty.
3. Understanding the economic, educational, and other social characteristics of Mexican-Americans requires a basic knowledge of traditional and nontraditional lifestyles.
B. Traditional Mexican-American families
1. The family is a close-knit group in which elders are the decision makers.
2. Extended family members often live with the nuclear family.
3. All family members regard the family as the main focus of social identification, with each member being a symbol of the family.

4. It is within the family that one is disciplined and receives love and understanding.
5. If possible, the members of the family live in close proximity to each other and visit frequently.
6. The father is the unquestioned authority of the household.
   a. He is hard, unyielding, and strong and typically reflects a machismo demeanor.
   b. The family members show him respect at all times.
   c. It is his duty to care for the family as provider.
7. The mother is soft, nurturing, and self-sacrificing.
   a. Her place is in the home, ensuring that the household runs properly.
   b. She does not openly question her husband's actions.
8. The children are expected to contribute to the running of the household.
   a. The girls help the mother with chores.
   b. Boys typically find jobs as soon as they are old enough to contribute monetarily to the family.
C. Non-traditional Mexican-American families
1. The nontraditional Mexican-American family may have adopted patterns that are the result of migration into white communities to improve economic or educational levels.
2. Certain characteristics, such as close family ties, health beliefs, and recreational patterns, generally remain.

IV. **Beliefs of Disease Causation Among Mexican-Americans**
A. Mexican-Americans typically view health and disease as an area in which God or some other force has been influential, either directly or indirectly.
1. A particular illness may be a form of *castigos* (punishment imposed by the supernatural, usually God).
2. *Brujas* (witches) are a malevolent source of illness.
B. Folk healing (*curanderismo*) is very important in Mexican-American culture.
1. The *curandero,* or healer, is a diagnostician, counselor, or practitioner and has derived powers for healing from God.
2. Mexican-American folk medicine considers three types of causation.
   a. Empirical
   b. Magical
   c. Psychological

3. Folk medicine ascribes to "hot and cold" imbalance diseases, diseases caused by dislocation of internal organs, diseases of emotional origin, and diseases of magical origin. Sources of ill health include food, shock, accidents, bodily malfunction, age, abuse of the body, congenital anomalies, heredity, contact with the elements, contact with people, and occupational causes.

C. Diseases caused by dislocation of internal organs
1. *Caida de la mollera* is a disease of infants that occurs when the fontanel of the parietal or frontal bone of the cranium falls and leaves a "soft spot."
   a. This usually happens during breast-feeding or as a result of a sudden fall.
   b. Treatment consists of putting salt on the fallen fontanel and allowing it to remain for three days.
   c. The infant is usually spoon-fed during the illness, and normal feeding cannot be resumed until the fontanel has been raised to its normal position.
2. *Empacho* is an infirmity of both children and adults that occurs when food particles become lodged in the intestinal tract and cause sharp pains.
   a. *Empacho* is usually not a serious infirmity.
   b. To treat this problem, a person lies face down on a bed with the back bared, and the curer lifts a piece of skin from the waist and pinches it to dislodge the offending material.
   c. Herbs and drugs may be administered to penetrate, soften, and crumble the food.

D. Diseases of emotional origin—Many physical diseases are traced to emotional origins and are treated psychosomatically.
1. *Bilis* (bile) is based on the ancient Greek belief in the four humors.
   a. These humors must remain in balance for a person to enjoy good health.
   b. An emotional experience such as anger or fear may cause the humors to become unbalanced and excess bile to flow into the bloodstream.
   c. *Bilis* is ordinarily treated with herbal remedies.
2. *Susto* (fright sickness) is very common in Mexico; an unexpected disturbing or emotional experience may cause *susto*.

a. Symptoms include diarrhea, fever, vomiting, and anorexia; *susto* can be fatal.
b. *Susto* is attributed to a spirit loss.
c. The practitioner calls the spirit back into the patient's body to effect the cure.

E. Disease of magical origin—*mal ojo*
1. *Mal ojo* is assumed to be the magical origin of many illnesses, especially those affecting children.
2. Infants with *mal ojo* sleep restlessly, cry for no apparent reason, are feverish, and have vomiting and diarrhea.
3. It is treated by rubbing the body with an egg for three consecutive evenings while chanting prayers. The egg will be broken and left overnight under the head of the bed. In the morning, if the egg appears to be "cooked" then *mal ojo* was the cause of the illness.
4. It is thought that *mal ojo* can be prevented by the use of *ojos de venado* (amulets) or red string or yarn tied around the wrist.

F. The hot-cold syndrome
1. Exposure to excessive heat or cold may be the main cause of illness.
2. Certain foods are thought to cause illness if they generate heat or cold within the body.
   a. Illnesses believed to be caused when *cold* enters the body are chest cramps, earache, headache, paralysis, sprains, stomach cramps, rheumatism, teething, and tuberculosis.
   b. Overabundance of *heat* in the body may cause dysentery, sore eyes, kidney ailments, abscessed teeth, sore throat, warts, and rashes.

V. **Use of Herbal Medicine**
A. Plant remedies are the most universal form of treatment.
B. Among Mexican-Americans, herbal medicine has strong cultural and historical ties to Indian, Aztec, and Spanish-Moorish societies.
C. Herbs may be used in combination with prayer and touch.
D. The use of herbs in combination with prayer and touch is seen in a variety of rituals associated with folk illnesses such as *susto* and *mal ojo*.
E. Medicinal herbs and the conditions they treat
1. Rattlesnake oil—rheumatism
2. Mineral water—kidney stones
3. Garlic—diphtheria prevention, pain in the bowels, toothache, rabid dog bite, stomach trouble, snakebite, hypertension

4. Cottonwood—swollen gums, ulcerated tooth, boils, broken bones
5. Sweet basil—hornet bite, colic
6. Apricot—goiter, dryness of the nose
7. Camphor—pain, rheumatism, headache, faintness
8. Alfalfa—bed bugs
9. Lavender—phlegm, colic, vomiting, menopause
10. Licorice—clotted blood
11. Parsley—painful shoulders, colic, stomach troubles
12. Wild pitplant—pyorrhea, throat irritation, skin irritation
13. Desert tea—headaches, cold, fever, kidney pain
14. Scouring brush—gonorrhea
15. Spearmint—female troubles, childbirth, newborns, colic, and menstrual cramps

F. Nurses should not be critical of the practice of herbal medicine but recognize it as an alternative health care that supplements modern medical practice.

G. Nurses usually should allow patients to continue their herbal regimen, but at the same time encourage the use of modern medical care and practice.

VI. **Cultural Adaptation to Health Care**
A. Improving access
1. Because of a lower economic level, certain conveniences, such as transportation and telephones, may not be available to many Mexican-Americans.
2. This produces problems such as access to health care.
3. Improving access to health care for Mexican-Americans may include having satellite clinics in the community, making appointment times more convenient (including evening and weekend hours), or working through neigh-borhood associations and churches to provide care and health education. Mobile vans are used as portable treatment facilities in some communities.
B. Reducing language barriers and improving communication
1. Mexican-American folk medicine is a matter of personal relations, familiar procedures, active family participation, home care, and control of the situation by the patient or family. In contrast, scientific medicine is impersonal and unfamiliar, gives control of the situation to the health care providers, and requires passivity from the family members. These differences create communication problems.
2. Communication between practitioners and patients should be dialogue-based rather than consisting of one-sided imperatives.
a. This is particularly important because the patient and practitioner may not use the same words for the same meanings of the disease process.
b. The use of bilingual and bicultural health practitioners should be encouraged whenever possible.

VII. **Improving Health Education and Communication**
A. Health promotion messages and health care to Hispanic groups are most effective when delivered within their social frame of reference and focus on problems known to exist in the community.
B. Success is enhanced when the following conditions are satisfied.
1. There is community involvement and outreach.
2. Programs focus on comprehensive services, including disease prevention and health promotion.
3. Cultural sensitivity is in evidence.
4. Access to health services is improved by the program.

TEACHING STRATEGIES

1. Invite a Mexican-American nurse to speak to the class. Have the nurse discuss folk healing and other cultural beliefs and practices. What can all nurses to do improve health care to this aggregate? How can nurses be more culturally sensitive?
2. Have a group of students review census data to identify the percentage of people of Hispanic origin in the local community. Delineate the various countries of origin for Hispanics. If possible, compare to previous data. Has the percentage increased since 1980? Since 1990? What are projections for the future?

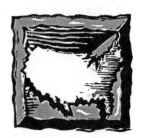

Cultural Influences in the Community: Other Populations

LEARNING OBJECTIVES

1. Identify a diverse population.

2. Describe three methods of assessing a diverse population within the community.

3. Compare and contrast the three methods of assessing a diverse population within the community.

4. Discuss the theoretical bases for program planning, implementation, and evaluation following the needs assessment of your population.

5. Identify a vulnerable population.

6. Discuss the seven properties of a vulnerable population.

7. Apply two implications for conducting research from the use of the guiding concept—marginalization— to a needs assessment of a diverse population.

LECTURE NOTES

Chapter 20 comprises five reprinted articles about diverse populations in the United States. In addition to supplying information about specific groups, the articles encourage students to refer to original articles for cultural information and introduce them to several journals that will be useful as future sources.

The articles introduce various approaches to community assessment and interventions for diverse populations. In many communities, assessment of a diverse population may not exist; in these cases, an assessment must be generated by the student in the community. Government vital and health statistics generally exist only for mainstream minority populations.

Students may need to assess a diverse population in a community, such as an immigrant group, to determine

the health status and needs of the community. Models used to approach an assessment of a population in the community are presented in the following chapters and include:

- the use of routinely reported data (vital statistics and communicable disease reports). D.C. Grossman et al., "Health status of urban American Indians and Alaska Natives." *JAMA* 271:845-850 (1994).

- extensive manual and computer-based searches of government and private sources of information, with specific techniques for uncovering information that is difficult to locate about a diverse community. M.S. Chen, Jr., B.L. Hawks, "A debunking of the myth of healthy Asian Americans and Pacific Islanders." *Am J Health Promotion* 19:261-268 (1995).

- conducting a needs assessment, including demographic, ethnographic, and historical information about a population in its social and geographical setting, as well as program planning, implementation, and evaluation based on the needs assessment. A.I. Meleis, P.A. Omidian, and J.G. Lipson, "Women's health status in the United States: An immigrant women's project," in *Women's Health and Development: A Global Challenge*, ed. B.J. McElmurry, K.F. Norr, and R.S. Parker (Boston: Jones and Bartlett, 1993), 163-181; M.A. Muecke, "Cultural influence in the community: Southeast Asian refugees." *American Journal of Public Health* 73, no. 4 (April 1983).

- the presentation of a concept—marginalization— and its properties to encourage the reader to examine implications for shaping nursing research, theory, and practice related to the health of vulnerable populations. J.M. Hall, P.E. Stevens, and A.I. Meleis, "Marginalization: A guiding concept for valuing diversity in nursing knowledge development." *Adv Nurs Sci* 16:23-41 (1994).

The student is encouraged to engage in the process of critical thinking by identifying vulnerable populations in the community; developing an approach to assessing the needs of the populations; carrying out the assessment; and engaging in program planning, implementation, and evaluation based on the assessment.

LEARNING ACTIVITIES

The learning activities listed here can be applied across the articles and aggregates discussed in the chapter.

1. Identify a vulnerable population within your community; discuss two properties that make this population vulnerable.

2. Identify a diverse population within your community for which traditional health indicators such as longevity, mortality, morbidity, and health services usage are not readily known.

3. Design an approach for assessment of a diverse population within your community. What data are available? What data would you need to collect that are not readily available?

4. Conduct an assessment of the diverse population you identified within your community.

5. Based on the needs assessment of the diverse population you identified in your community, design a program plan, an implementation plan, and an evaluation.

6. List two implications from the use of the guiding concept of marginalization for valuing the diversity in your selected population; state how the choice of a relevant design, sampling at the margins, and reflexive involvement of the marginalized people or groups in your population can be applied in the development of your assessment and program.

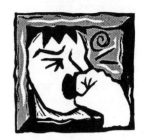

Violence in the Community

ANNOTATED LEARNING OBJECTIVES

1. Describe the concept of community violence.

The term *violence* refers to any behaviors that cause injury or death. Community violence has been declared a public health epidemic and has been identified as a worse health problem for women and children than cancer. Many social and economic factors (poverty, racism, disintegration of the family, etc.) contribute to violence. It is important to realize that violence is a learned behavior and can be changed and prevented.

2. Identify the long-term effects of violence on our society.

Child abuse accounts for hundreds of deaths each year. In 1985, almost 2000 cases were reported per 10,000 children. Many of these were neglect.

Long-term problems include perpetuation of the violent cycle, emotional and physical scars, lowered self-esteem, addiction to narcotics, developmental and mental delays, and failure to thrive.

In addition to physical and emotional pain, spouse abuse can cause diminished self-esteem, isolation, and loss of an unborn baby. Spouse abuse accounts for the deaths of hundreds of women and men each year in the United States.

Domestic violence is cyclic; women and men who were exposed to abuse as children tend to repeat the process. Elder abuse may become more prevalent as citizens live longer. Long-term effects include diminished respect for life of elders and failure to respect their rights and needs.

3. Identify the effect of guns on the problem of violence.

During the 1980s, almost three times as many people died from gunshot wounds as died from

AIDS, and guns killed more than five times the number of Americans killed during the Vietnam War. On an average day, more than 700 Americans are shot, and 65 of those shot die. Seventy-five percent of homicide victims and more than 50% of suicide victims die of gunshot wounds. Although guns do not cause violence, they greatly raise the severity of the health consequences. It is estimated that 20–25% of nonfatal gunshot wounds cause permanent impairment. Finally, the economic costs associated with gun-related violence are staggering.

4. Identify populations at risk for violence and the role of public health in dealing with the epidemic of violence.

Those at risk for violence include youth, women (particularly pregnant women), children, and elders. Other contributing factors include availability of guns, history of family violence, poverty, use of drugs/alcohol, media violence, and gang involvement.

A number of public health efforts have been taken recently to control the problem of violence. Violence has been termed a public health epidemic in the United States. To address the issue of violence, 18 of the objectives of *Healthy People 2000* are related to reduction of violence. Specific goals and suggestions for meeting these goals have been developed, and community leaders and health care providers are encouraged to work together to implement programs to reach the identified goals.

5. Analyze assessment data to determine the risk of abuse.

Child abuse is more common when the parents abuse drugs or alcohol and when the parents were raised in homes where physical, emotional, or sexual abuse was practiced. The nurse should be alert for signs of physical and emotional abuse and neglect (unexplained bruises, burns, fractures, consistent hunger, poor hygiene, lack of medical care). The nurse should observe the parent's behavior with the child and the child's with the parent.

Nurses working in primary care areas should be alert to repeated or unexplained injuries in women clients. Women clients who have expressed fear of their spouses, or who report substance abuse, may be at risk.

Likewise, elders who have unexplained physical injuries or evidence of restraint or repeatedly appear unkempt or neglected may be victims. The primary caregivers may report stress in the situation.

6. *Describe the role of the nurse in primary, secondary, and tertiary prevention of violence.*

Primary prevention of abuse includes promotion of family strengths. Education on violence and long-term effects should begin in elementary school and should increase awareness of abusive patterns. Primary prevention focuses on the improvement of parent-child, husband-wife, and caregiver-elder relationship. Parenting education can be a useful means to decrease child abuse. Altering social attitudes to decrease acceptance of domestic violence and identification of women at risk can decrease the abuse of women. The nurse should work with caregivers of the elderly to decrease stress. Provision of respite care or home health aides may decrease elder abuse.

Secondary prevention focuses on recognition of signs and symptoms of abuse and appropriately treats both physical and psychological problems on the individual, family, and community levels. Legal intervention may be necessary at this level.

Tertiary prevention efforts should be directed to long-term psychological treatment of the abused and the abuser. Group therapy and counseling can help overcome long-term psychological problems and ultimately break the abuse cycle.

7. *Identify protection measures necessary for nurses working in situations where violence is prevalent.*

When working in places where violence is prevalent, the nurse should be aware of threats, risks and potentially harmful situations. Identification of risk factors and high-risk situations may offer some protection. The nurse who works in the community must be very aware of the environment. To promote safety, the nurse should plan ahead (know the area, schedule a visit ahead of time, inform the office, dress for function, wear a name tag, drive a trustworthy vehicle); approach the home carefully(note animals, fences, activity, indicators of crime, listen for signs of fighting or feelings of unease); be aware of who is in the home; and note exits. The nurse should leave and call 911 if violence occurs.

LECTURE OUTLINE

Violence has been declared a public health epidemic and has been identified as a worse health problem for women and children than cancer. The term violence *refers to any behaviors that cause injury or death. Many social and economic factors (poverty, racism, disintegration of the family, etc.) contribute to violence. It is important to realize that violence is a learned behavior and that it can be changed and prevented.*

I. **History of Abuse**
A. Humans have dealt with other humans violently since the beginning of time.
B. Infanticide has been practiced throughout history.
   1. Children were sacrificed for religious reasons.
   2. A sickly or deformed child, a twin, or a girl was sometimes left to die from exposure or by some other means.
C. Corporal punishment has been a means of controlling children through the ages.
D. Historically, wives were considered the property of their husbands, and wife beating was legal in the United States until 1824.
E. Elder abuse has recently been recognized as a growing problem, although it is not unique to the 20th century. The problem is of greater magnitude today because people are living longer, so there are more elderly people.

II. **Scope of the Problem**
A. Homicide
   1. America is the most violent country in the industrialized world. The number of deaths by violence in the United States exceeds the combined total of the next 17 nations.
   2. Homicide is the tenth leading cause of death among all age groups.
   3. At risk for homicide are young people, women, and African-American and Hispanic males.
   4. Homicide is the second leading cause of death among Americans ages 15–24 and the leading cause of death among African-American males ages 15–34.
   5. Because of increases in violent crime among teens, government officials have warned that more importance must be given to preventing young people from becoming criminals.

6. Homicide is the fourth leading cause of death from injury among females, disproportionately affecting African-American females.

B. Suicide
   1. Suicide is the eighth leading cause of death in all age groups in the United States, and rates appear to be increasing.
   2. Guns are used in 60% of teen suicides.
   3. Depression and impulsiveness are risk factors for suicide, particularly among teens and young adults.

C. Assault
   1. Assault, primarily in the context of marital or dating relationships, is a major source of injury to females.
   2. It is reported that 22–35% of all women seeking treatment in emergency rooms are abused.

D. Impact of guns
   1. It is interesting to note that during the 1980s, almost three times as many people died from gunshot wounds as died from AIDS, and guns killed more than five times the number of Americans killed during the Vietnam War.
   2. On an average day, more than 700 Americans are shot; 65 of those shot die.
   3. Seventy-five percent of homicide victims and more than 50% of suicide victims die of gunshot wounds.

III. **Violence of Aggregates**
A. Youth-related violence
   1. Violent crimes among youth are increasing, and crimes such as homicide, rape, robbery, and aggravated assault are much more prevalent among adolescents than among adults.
   2. Almost 50% of nonfatal crimes of violence in the United States are committed by people between the ages of 12 and 24.
   3. Minority youth are particularly affected.
   4. Risk factors for youth-related violence include repeated exposure to violence, drugs, easy access to firearms, unstable family life, poverty, family violence, delinquent peer groups, and media violence.

B. Domestic violence
   1. *Domestic violence* refers to a pattern of coercive behaviors that are perpetrated by someone who is, or was, in an intimate relationship with the victim. These behaviors include battering, psychological abuse, and sexual assault.
   2. Abuse is repetitive and often escalates in frequency and severity.
   3. Current estimates are that 2 to 4 million domestic partners are victims of abuse each year, although the scope of the problem is difficult to assess due to the large number of women who do not report the incidents.
   4. Domestic violence against women may be the single most common cause of injury in women presenting to the health care system.
   5. Battering of a man by a woman does occur, but the incidence is so low that it does not appear to be a significant health problem.
   6. Domestic abuse frequently begins or escalates during pregnancy.
      a. The results of violence include spontaneous abortion, stillbirths, and preterm deliveries.
      b. As a result, some authorities recommend that all pregnant women be screened for abuse.
   7. The cycle theory of violence explains that the pattern of violence contains three phases: tension, explosion, and contrition.
   8. The objective of the abuser is to exert power and control over the victim.
   9. Domestic violence includes emotional abuse and intimidation, minimizing, denying and blaming, coercion and threats, isolation, and economic abuse.
   10. The effects of repeated battering contribute to shock, denial confusion, withdrawal, psychological numbness, and fear.
      a. Fear and helplessness are the main reasons many women do not leave an abusive situation.
      b. Culture, religion, and economics are also factors.
      c. Those most likely to leave a battering situation are women who have resources (money, family, friends); have power; have no children; were not abused as children; did not see their mothers beaten; are involved in batterings that are frequent or severe; or have a partner who begins to beat children.

C. Child abuse—Child abuse is a socially learned behavior and is generational. There are four basic types of child abuse: physical abuse; neglect (both physical and emotional); emotional maltreatment; and sexual abuse.
   1. *Physical abuse* is a non-accidental physical injury that is inflicted on a child by another person.

a. Beating with an instrument is the most common type of physical abuse.

b. Cuts, bruises, burns, and fractures are the result.

c. Children ages 2–5 are the most frequently injured, but infants are in the greatest danger of severe injury or death (50% of fatalities were in infants less that one year old).

d. "Shaken baby syndrome" refers to violent shaking of a baby and can cause trauma at the brain stem-spinal cord junction.

   1) Serious and often permanent damage may occur.

   2) Men (mother's spouse or boyfriend) and baby-sitters are the people who most commonly inflict this type of injury.

2. *Child neglect* (physical and emotional) is negligent treatment or maltreatment of a child by a person responsible for the child's welfare.

a. Physical neglect is the failure to provide basic needs, including safety, food, clothing, shelter and health needs.

b. Emotional neglect is the lack of sensitivity and love shown by the parent for the child.

3. *Emotional maltreatment* is willful infliction of unjustifiable mental suffering, causing emotional damage.

a. Emotional maltreatment includes mental injury or commission of acts that might affect the child's normal emotional development.

b. Examples of emotional abuse include locking a child in a closet for a prolonged period of time, tying a child to a bedpost, or repeated name calling.

4. *Sexual abuse* is sexual activity between an adult and child.

a. Sexual abuse includes use of a child for sexual exploitation, prostitution, or pornography.

b. Incest is defined as sexual relations between close family members such as a father and daughter or siblings within the family.

c. Sexual abuse may occur over a prolonged period of time and involve threats to the child to continue the abuse.

d. Effects are often long-term.

e. Women who were sexually abused as children often suffer from depression, anxiety, and low self-esteem, and they experience sexual problems as adults.

5. Physical indicators of child abuse

a. Unexplained bruises and welts in various stages of healing

b. Unexplained burns by cigarettes, immersion burns, or rope burns

c. Unexplained lacerations or abrasions

d. Unexplained fractures

e. Unexplained injuries to mouth, lips, gums, eyes, or external genitalia.

f. Wariness of adults

g. Apprehensiveness when other children cry

h. Constantly on the alert for danger

i. Frightened of parents

j. Afraid to go home

6. Indicators of physical neglect

a. Hunger

b. Poor hygiene

c. Inappropriate dress

d. Lack of supervision

e. Lack of medical or dental care

f. Fatigue

g. Begging or stealing food

h. Stealing

i. Delinquency and/or early arrival and late departure from school

7. Indicators of sexual abuse

a. Difficulty in walking or sitting

b. Torn, stained, or bloody underwear

c. Genital pain or itching

d. Bruises or bleeding from the external genitalia, vagina, or anal area

e. Sexually transmitted disease

f. Drug and alcohol abuse

g. Developmental delays

h. Teen pregnancy

i. Negative self-esteem

j. Deficits in personal and social skills

k. Bizarre, sophisticated, or unusual sexual behavior or knowledge

l. Suicide ideation

m. Delinquency

n. Tendency to run away

8. Indicators of emotional maltreatment

a. Failure to thrive

b. Lagging in physical development

c. Speech disorders

d. Developmental delays

e. Behavior extremes from passivity to aggression

f. Habit and conduct disorders

g. Attempted suicide

D. Abuse of the elderly

1. Characteristics of elder abuse

a. *Elder abuse* refers any act or omission by a caregiver, guardian, or custodian of an elderly person which results in harm or threatened harm to that person's health or welfare.

b. It is estimated that between 1–10% of elders suffer some form of maltreatment.

c. The abuser is usually a member of the victim's family, most often one of their children (usually a son if the abuse is physical, a daughter if the abuse is emotional neglect or deprivation of rights, or either if the abuse is financial) who reside in the same household.

d. Grandchildren, spouses, and siblings can also be abusers.

e. A woman living with a male relative is at the greatest risk for abuse.

2. There are five commonly described types of abuse of the elderly.

a. Physical abuse—infliction of pain or injury, unnecessary physical restraining

b. Psychological or emotional abuse—verbal assault, threats, provoking fear, or isolation

c. Sexual abuse—unwanted sexual contact

d. Physical neglect—withholding personal care, food, medications or medical care, or lack of supervision

e. Financial exploitation—theft and misuse of money or property

3. Indicators of abuse

a. Physical indicators of elder abuse include injury that has not received care; cuts, lacerations, or puncture wounds; bruises; dehydration or loss of weight without illness-related cause; evidence of inadequate care or administration of medicine; poor skin hygiene; soiled clothing or bed; burns; and signs of confinement.

b. Behavioral indicators of elder abuse include fear, withdrawal, depression, helplessness, implausible stories, confusion, anger, denial, and agitation.

c. Financial indicators include refusal to spend money on the elder; recent will when the person is incapable of making a will; personal belongings missing; signatures on checks that do not resemble the elder's signature; and unusual activity in bank accounts.

d. Family/caregiver indicators of possible elder abuse include aggressive behavior; indifference or anger toward the elder; previous history of abuse to others; problems with alcohol or drugs; conflicting accounts of incidents by the family and victim; and restriction of the activity of the elder within the family unit.

IV. **Public Health Perspective**

A. Violence has been termed a public health epidemic in the United States.

B. To address the issue of violence and reduce its occurrence, 18 violence-related objectives of *Healthy People 2000* were identified.

C. Specific goals and suggestions for meeting these goals have been developed, and community leaders and health care providers are encouraged to work together to implement programs to reach the identified goals.

V. **Prevention of Violence in the Community**

A. Primary prevention should focus on promotion of family wellness.

1. Education, beginning in elementary school, should increase awareness of the problem of violence, facilitate case detection, and provide for early treatment.

2. Provision of community services to provide care for families before serious injury occurs is also key.

3. Reduction of violence in the media, control of handguns and assault weapons, working to change attitudes toward violence against women, education about parenting, and support for caregivers of the elderly are examples of primary prevention interventions.

B. Secondary prevention supports families in stress to facilitate early diagnosis and treatment.

1. Access to assistance must be around-the-clock.

2. Access to shelters and legal options is crucial.

3. Assessment of women during pregnancy is important.

4. Once a violent situation is known, the victim must be helped to plan for safety.

5. In cases of child or elder abuse, the nurse may be the one to report the injury to the authorities.

C. Tertiary prevention provides rehabilitative services to violent families.
 1. A social service agency or local law enforcement members should be involved.
 2. The abuser may be prosecuted and punished.
 3. Professional counseling and self-help groups can be helpful.

VI. Safety of the Health Professional
 A. The nurse is not immune to danger.
 B. Identification of risk factors and high-risk situations may offer some protection.
 C. The nurse who works in the community must be very aware of the environment.
 D. To promote safety, the nurse should take the following basic precautions.
  1. Plan ahead
   a. Know the area
   b. Schedule a visit ahead of time
   c. Inform the office
   d. Dress for function
   e. Wear a name tag
   f. Drive a trustworthy vehicle
  2. Approach the home carefully
   a. Note animals, fences, activity, and indicators of crime
   b. Listen for signs of fighting
   c. Note feelings of unease
  3. Be aware of who is in the home
  4. Note exits
  5. Leave and call 911 if violence occurs

VII. Nursing Diagnoses for Victims of Abuse—Nursing diagnoses appropriate for victims of abuse include anxiety, alteration in family process, hopelessness, knowledge deficit, powerlessness, post-trauma response, social isolation, and potential for violence.

TEACHING STRATEGIES

1. Invite a speaker from the local or regional child protective services to discuss child abuse. Request copies of the state's regulations for mandatory report of suspected abuse.
2. Invite a speaker from a battered women's shelter to discuss domestic violence. Have the speaker address issues of legal recourse for the victim and how to counsel victims of domestic violence.
3. Discuss the *Healthy People 2000* objectives dealing with "Violent and Abusive Behaviors." What, if any, progress has been made toward meeting these objectives? What can community health nurses do?
4. In groups of 3 or 4, have students practice completing the "Planning for Safety" checklist (Table 21–7). Encourage student discussion on how/when a tool of this sort should be used. What other interventions should nurses be prepared to make?
5. Discuss "Safety Issues for the Caregiver" (Table 21–9). Ensure that all students are aware of these issues and understand how to avoid and respond to threats of violence.

CHAPTER 22

Mental Health

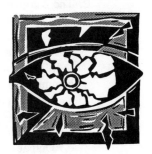

ANNOTATED LEARNING OBJECTIVES

1. *Describe the concept of aggregate mental health.*

   Aggregate mental health is the degree to which families and groups contribute to enhance or intensify individual interaction along the mental health/mental illness continuum within a given environment. Interventions for aggregate mental health emphasize community practice rather than treatment of mental illness in institutional settings. Services are offered within the context of community values, norms, and agencies.

2. *Describe how the nursing process is applied to promote the mental health of individuals and families in the community.*

   The nursing process serves as an organizing framework around which interventions to address aggregate mental health can be planned. Assessment of community mental health in aggregates involves identification of the community systems that comprise the aggregate and the boundaries.

   Using a deductive approach, the nurse can begin with assessment of the aggregate or community and apply the data to individuals and families. Using the inductive approach, assessment begins with the individual client and is followed by assessment of the family, aggregate, and community. Diagnoses should be written to address the actual and potential needs of the individual, family, aggregate, and community.

   Planning should involve goal setting between the nurse and client and should encompass all levels of prevention. Interventions should be based on these long- and short-term goals.

   Evaluation should be ongoing and should focus on achieving planned primary, secondary and tertiary interventions.

LECTURE OUTLINE

I. **Mental Health**
   A. Components of mental health for individuals
      1. The absence of mental disease
      2. Normality of behavior
      3. Adjustment to environment
      4. Unity of personality
      5. Correct perception of reality
   B. When people experience mental illness, abnormal behavior, environmental maladjustment, disunity of personality, or altered perceptions of reality, the family or group to which the individual belongs is also affected.
   C. Aggregate mental health is the degree to which families and groups contribute to enhance or intensify individual interaction along the mental health/mental illness continuum within a given environment.

II. **Community Mental Health Movement**
   A. Characteristics of community mental health
      1. Community mental health emphasizes community practice rather than treatment of mental illness in institutional settings.
      2. It acknowledges the importance of offering services within the context of community values, norms, and agencies.
   B. The three phases of psychiatric evolution
      1. The independent science phase, at the end of the 18th century, stressed an empathic attitude toward mental illness.
      2. In the late 19th century, Sigmund Freud developed psychoanalysis.
      3. The phase of community psychiatry, which began in the 1960s, emphasized community care rather than treatment in institutional settings.

C. Legislation
1. The *Community Mental Health Centers Construction Act of 1963* was the result of concern about the quality of mental health care. This act established community-based therapeutic centers to replace custodial mental institutions.
2. The *National Institutes of Mental Health* were established in the early 1960s to address mental health promotion and maintenance. The National Institute of Mental Health (NIMH) identified the essential elements of community mental health services.
   a. Inpatient services
   b. Partial hospitalization or at least day care service
   c. Outpatient services
   d. Emergency services on a 24-hour basis
   e. Consultation and educational services available to community agencies and professionals
3. The *Community Mental Health Centers Amendments* (1975) increased the number of essential services required of community mental health centers.
4. The *Omnibus Budget Reconciliation Act* and the repeal of Community Mental Health Systems Act in the early 1980s produced financial cutbacks that have impeded most programs.

III. **Factors Contributing to the Mental Health of Aggregates**
A. Environmental factors
1. Environmental factors that affect mental health include lead poisoning, other heavy metal poisoning, pesticide poisoning, carbon monoxide poisoning, and acute chemical poisoning.
2. When aggregates are exposed to toxins, the functioning of the entire community may be hindered.
B. Biological factors—Regular physical activity benefits mental health by managing depression and anxiety.
C. Social factors
1. Psychosocial interventions can improve psychological well-being during life conditions by enhancing social supports systems and by strengthening an individual's interpersonal, psychological, and physical resources.
2. A number of *Healthy People 2000* objectives address social factors that affect mental health.

IV. **Assessment of Aggregate Mental Health**—Assessment of aggregate mental health should integrate application of systems theory, the nursing process, and a theoretical approach for analysis of groups and families.
A. Nursing process
1. Good observational skills and the use of therapeutic communication are important in assessing aggregate mental health.
2. The nurse must look beyond the individual client to consider the family or social groups, environment, and society when addressing community mental health issues.
3. An understanding of group processes and group analysis is helpful.
B. Roles of the community mental health nurse
1. Educator
   a. As an educator, the nurse instructs individuals, families and/or groups about various aspects of preventive mental health; treatment of mental illness; and management of individuals who are mentally ill, yet function in the community.
   b. Group and family education provides a support network for exchange of ideas related to illness management and allows people to share their feelings about the impact of the illness.
2. Practitioner
   a. As a practitioner, the nurse forms a therapeutic relationship with individuals, groups, and families and then works with them directly.
   b. Provision of individual, group, and family therapy by an advanced practitioner facilitates the mental health of aggregates by identifying those dynamics that interfere with or enhance the person's experience with the environment and the mental illness.
   c. Reasons for referral to community health nurses include discharge follow-up, assessment, medication monitoring, crisis intervention, parent education, and prevention.
3. Coordinator
   a. The community mental health nurse receives referrals from a variety of sources.
   b. As coordinator, the nurse refers clients to other professionals, including social workers, psychologists, psychiatrists, occupational therapists, physical therapists, and speech therapists.

C. Phases of the therapeutic relationship
1. Initial phase
   a. Client and nurse get to know each other.
   b. Together, they identify client needs and create a contract to specify the responsibilities of the nurse and the client in goal attainment.
   c. They formulate nursing diagnoses to reflect mutually identified problems and needs of the client, whether individual, family, group, or community.
2. Working phase
   a. Identification of patterns of behavior that cause disequilibrium
   b. Identification of intrapersonal, interpersonal, and other system components that may be detrimental to mental health
   c. Exploration of ways to modify dysfunctional behavior patterns
   d. Testing new and modified patterns
   e. Identification of problematic client/ nurse/system boundary issues.
3. Termination phase
   a. The nurse and client summarize the outcomes of the relationship.
   b. They explore the extent of goal achievement.
   c. They identify plans for continuity of care.

V. **Application of the Nursing Process to Community Mental Health**
A. Assessment
1. Assessment of aggregates in community mental health involves identifying the community systems that comprise the aggregate and the boundaries of those systems. The boundaries may be cultural, ethnic, geographical, socioeconomic, or religious.
2. When assessing community mental health, the nurse might use a deductive approach.
   a. The deductive approach begins with the community's concept of mental health/ mental illness and work toward the individuals, families, and groups that make up that community.
   b. The deductive approach starts with a community study to identify groups at high risk for mental illness, families in crisis, and individuals having difficulty coping with activities of daily living.
3. The nurse can also use an inductive approach to assess community mental health.
   a. The nurse begins by assessing the individual as client.

b. To assess the individual, the nurse must identify the family, groups, and community to which the person belongs and then assess them also.
B. Diagnosis
1. Nursing diagnoses should be written for the actual and potential needs of the individual, family, aggregate, and community.
2. A diagnosis can be made for each system component, leading to an aggregate diagnosis.
   a. An example of an *individual* nursing diagnosis is: "Decreased ability to perform activities of daily living related to self-discontinuance of antipsychotic medication."
   b. An example of a *family* nursing diagnosis is: "Potential family crises related to decreased equilibrium."
   c. An example of a *community* nursing diagnosis is: "Lack of understanding related to inadequate information about schizophrenia."
C. Planning
1. Planning typically involves contracting with aggregates to establish care.
2. Mutual goal setting through collaboration with the agent and clientele is essential during the planning phase.
3. Plans may include intervention at the primary, secondary and/or tertiary levels.
D. Intervention
1. Interventions based on individual, family, aggregate and community long- and short-term goals are implemented.
2. Alternative interventions are planned and implemented, if possible, if those originally planned are not successful.
E. Evaluation
1. Evaluation by the nurse should be ongoing and multidimensional, including components of the individual, family, aggregate, and community systems.
2. Evaluation of nursing intervention should include goal achievement of planned primary, secondary, and tertiary interventions.
3. Major points of nursing intervention that should be evaluated include
   a. Health education
   b. Drug supervision
   c. Counseling
   d. Family therapy
   e. Behavior therapy
   f. Referral

TEACHING STRATEGIES

1. Invite a community mental health nurse to speak to the class. Have the nurse explain various aspects of practice, including sources of patient referrals, various roles performed, and legislation and funding for mental health.

2. Divide the class into groups of 2 or 3 students. Assign each group to identify, investigate, and visit area organizations and providers that care for people with mental disorders or work to improve mental health. With the entire class, have each group share what they discovered. Questions to address include: What services are available? What services are minimal, lacking or overcrowded? How are services accessed? What interventions are provided? What are responsibilities of nurses in these organizations or agencies?

CHAPTER 23

Substance Abuse

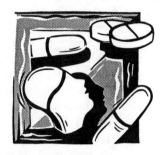

ANNOTATED LEARNING OBJECTIVES

1. Discuss the historical trends and current conceptions of the cause and treatment of substance abuse.

Historically, medical models have described substance abuse as an individual malfunction that involves the loss of control over drinking or the use of legal or illegal drugs. Genetic risk has been implicated in development of addiction. Currently, multicausal models are accepted as the source of development of substance abuse and dependency.

Treatment for substance abuse problems should be multifaceted to address the multiple contributing factors. Education to recognize and prevent substance use and abuse is essential. Treatment consists of a combination of strategies, including management of detoxification, group and/or individual therapy, counseling, aversion therapy, hypnosis, mutual help groups, psychoanalysis, and other approaches.

2. Describe the current social, political, and economic aspects of substance abuse.

Because of cultural differences, substance abuse problems may be difficult to identify. Social difficulties such as racism, unemployment, poverty, lack of role models, and peer pressure increase the possibility of use and abuse of potentially addictive substances.

Legislative or political interventions attempt to limit access and use of potentially addictive substances. In the United States, laws have been adopted to restrict alcohol use by minors, eliminate driving while intoxicated, prohibit smoking on airlines, and control illegal drugs in an attempt to reduce the incidence of substance abuse.

Economics influence substance abuse in a number of ways. Poverty and related difficulties often result in the use of drugs in an attempt to cope with problems. The individual's economic situation and role models can pressure or encourage the individual to use and sell illegal substances. Use of legal drugs such as alcohol and nicotine are encouraged by media marketing campaigns, which depict their use as desirable.

3. Identify issues related to substance abuse in various populations encountered in community health nursing practice.

Women, particularly those who are non-white and have a low income, are vulnerable to abusing drugs. The chemical effects of drugs seems to be more pronounced in women, causing more medical problems, faster intoxication, and more rapid progression of alcoholism. African-Americans, Hispanics, and Native Americans are thought to be especially at risk for development of problems with substance abuse. Adolescents may develop substance abuse patterns due to the combined influences of peer pressure, physiological immaturity, social role pressures, risk-taking orientation, and the lack of other recreational alternatives. The elderly may be vulnerable to problems because of diminished physiological tolerance, increased use of medically prescribed drugs, and effects of social isolation.

4. Detail the typical symptoms and consequences of substance abuse.

Typically, an individual begins with social use of drugs or alcohol. Initial exposures may be either pleasant and reinforcing or unpleasant. Social use may continue for a while; at this stage, the individual does not appear to have any detrimental effects from the substance. The individual has control, but use becomes more frequent. This can be followed by progression to abuse if the substance is used more often and in more varied settings. Denial and rationalization for use are common. Periods of abstinence may occur during which the individual does not use the substance. Dependency or addiction is marked by an increasing focus on the substance and its procurement and a narrowing of interests, social activities, and relationships.

5. *Applying the nursing process to substance abuse problems presented in a case study.*

Assessment of individuals, families, and communities should be comprehensive. The nurse should collect data on possible abuse regardless of threat of embarrassment, being sensitive to clues from behavior and clues during home visits that might indicate substance dependency or abuse. Nursing diagnoses are based on assessment data and may include alteration in comfort related to withdrawal, self-care deficits, hopelessness, anxiety, feelings of powerlessness, alteration in nutrition, and social isolation.

Nursing roles for intervention include education, direct care provision, counseling, collaboration with other health care disciplines, coordination of services, and consultation. Evaluation is ongoing and is based on outcomes of interventions and goal attainment.

6. *Assess and describe the needs of special populations of substance abusers.*

Ethnic and racial minorities may be particularly susceptible to development of abuse patterns due to the combined effects of poverty, oppression, underemployment, decreased job opportunities, stress, culture values, and role models. Barriers to treatment of substance abuse in minority populations can include lack of available or accessible treatment programs, lifestyles that accept selling drugs, inadequate social support for recovery, diminished self-esteem due to racism, and easy access to alcohol and drugs.

Individuals diagnosed with substance abuse as well as other psychiatric diagnoses are said to have *dual diagnoses*. Individuals with dual diagnoses present several problems due to complicated treatment regimens and, frequently, problems with dysfunctional families.

Individuals who are HIV-positive present special problems related to high-risk behaviors and impairment of the immune system due to the effects of drugs and alcohol. Substance abuse also enhances the physical and mental deterioration caused by HIV. Finally, health care providers are vulnerable because of accessibility of drugs and work-related stress.

LECTURE OUTLINE

Substance abuse has many far-reaching consequences, including social, psychological, physical, economic, and political problems. In the United States, more illnesses and disabilities and deaths are attributed to substance abuse than any other preventable health condition. It is estimated that substance abuse costs approximately $240 billion annually.

I. **Historic Trends in the Use of Alcohol and Illicit Drugs**
   A. Shifts in public tolerance, political and economic trends, and other factors have influenced the fluctuations in the use of alcohol and illicit drugs in the United States.
      1. Alcohol consumption
         a. Consumption was high during both world wars, but decreased during Prohibition and the Great Depression.
         b. Alcohol use was highest around 1980, attributable to most states lowering the drinking age to 18 years.
         c. There has been a recent decline due to a shift in preference away from distilled beverages to wine and beer.
      2. Drug consumption
         a. In the 19th century, morphine was used to treat a variety of health problems, but at the beginning of the 20th century, concern over the addictive nature of opiates and cocaine led to government regulation.
         b. The Harrison Narcotic Act of 1914 (and subsequent laws) limited physicians' ability to prescribe and dispense addictive drugs and restricted importation of narcotics.
         c. During the 1960s, heroin use became a problem in the inner cities.
         d. By the 1970s, increased availability and a positive attitude toward drug use in young people caused the use of heroin and other drugs to spread.
         e. Drug use peaked around 1979.
         f. During the 1980s and 1990s, use of marijuana and most other drugs declined, but cocaine and "crack" cocaine have continued to be used by many adolescents and young adults.
   B. To combat illicit drug abuse and dependence, federal drug policy has emphasized law enforcement and efforts to reduce the supply. Recently, prevention and treatment programs have been implemented to decrease the amount

of illicit drugs used in the United States and to lessen their impact.

II. **Prevalence of Substance Abuse**
   A. Alcohol use—In a 1992 survey, 65% of Americans reported using alcohol in the past year, and 20% consume it once a week or more often.
   B. About 11% of the general United States population reported using illicit drugs in the past year, and 5.5% had used them in the last month.
      1. Marijuana was the most commonly used illicit drug, with 33% of the population reporting marijuana use during their lifetime and 4.4% using it currently.
      2. About 11% reported using cocaine in their lifetime, and .6% had used cocaine in the last month.

III. **Concepts of Substance Abuse**
   A. Definitions—The American Psychiatric Association has classified psychoactive substance abuse disorders as either dependence or abuse of any substance that affects the nervous system (psychoactive).
      1. *Dependence* criteria include cognitive, behavioral, and physiologic symptoms common to all categories of psychoactive substances. Symptoms indicate that the user has impaired control of the effect of the substance and continues to use it despite adverse consequences. The symptoms of dependence include physiologic tolerance and withdrawal. Dependence is classified by severity (mild, moderate, or severe), or the user can be in partial or full remission.
      2. Psychoactive substance *abuse* is not as severe as dependence and does not include tolerance and withdrawal, but does indicate maladaptive patterns of use. It is a precursor to substance dependence.
   B. Causes of substance abuse
      1. Theories of substance abuse may address individual physiologic, spiritual, and psychological factors or may deal with social influences such as family, ethnicity, race, access, environmental stressors, economics, culture, or sex roles.
      2. A combination of factors is generally cited as the underlying impetus for substance abuse.
   C. Sociocultural and political aspects of substance abuse
      1. Because of cultural differences, it may be difficult to determine when a substance abuse problem exists.
         a. Each subculture may socially define abuse in a different way.
         b. The expectations of what drugs will do are shaped by the culture of the user and involve the adoption of roles that are learned and reinforced by social groups.
      2. The ways in which drugs are produced and distributed among the various segments of the population are determined largely by economic, cultural, and political conditions.
   D. Crack cocaine epidemic—Sociocultural influences on substance abuse patterns can be illustrated by the crack cocaine epidemic.
      1. Cocaine abuse is currently at epidemic proportions, with an estimated 2.2 million Americans using cocaine at least weekly.
      2. The availability of cocaine has increased dramatically over the past decade, particularly in areas with high population density.
      3. Crack cocaine is the newest form of cocaine and is relatively inexpensive, allowing its use by adolescents, young adults, and the poor. As a result, poverty, unemployment, community disintegration, social and psychological isolation, and depression cannot be separated from the epidemic.
      4. The crisis is particularly evident in the African-American communities of many U.S. metropolitan areas.
      5. The concept of "intersecting epidemics" is applicable to crack cocaine use.
         a. The association between crack and STDs and HIV infection is related to bartering sex for drugs.
         b. Women addicted to crack are usually unable to stop drug use without treatment on becoming pregnant; therefore, complications such as risk of spontaneous abortion, premature delivery, and addicted babies are increasing.
   E. Typical course of addictive illness—Genetic and environmental vulnerabilities affect the progression from initiation to continuation, transition, abuse, addiction, and dependency.
      1. Social use stage
         a. Typically, the individual begins with social use of the substance.
         b. The initial exposure may be pleasant and reinforcing, or unpleasant enough to prevent further use.
         c. Cocaine most often produces strong feelings of euphoria, alertness, control, and increased energy, so future use is generally enticing.

2. Continuation stage—Substance use persists, but it does not appear to be detrimental to the individual.
3. Transition stage
   a. Individuals have some control over use, but use becomes more frequent.
   b. A binge pattern is often seen during the transition stage.
4. Abuse stage
   a. The abuse stage is evidenced by the use of the substance more often and in more varied settings.
   b. Rationalizations are commonly used to deny the seriousness and consequences of substance use.
   c. Use may be interspersed with periods of abstinence, which reinforces the individual's perceived sense of control over the substance use. In cocaine, addiction abstinence symptoms include depression, lethargy, and inability to feel pleasure. Withdrawal can result in depression.
5. Addiction or dependency stage
   a. Development of the addiction or dependency stage is marked by an increasing focus on the substance and a narrowing of interests, social activities, and relationships.
   b. The individual becomes preoccupied with the substance and its procurement.

IV. **Modes of Intervention**
   A. Overview
      1. Prevention is critical in minimizing the impact of alcohol and drug problems on contemporary society. At the federal level, prevention efforts have been overshadowed by the "war on drugs." A great deal of money has been allocated to law enforcement, interdiction, crop eradication, and harsh laws to prosecute drug users and manufacturers.
      2. There is some debate about the potential benefits of legalization and decriminalization and the impact they would have on individuals and society.
         a. Arguments supporting legalization and decriminalization include a reduction in crime and moving the drug problem out of "moral failing" and toward humane treatment.
         b. Opposing arguments include the belief that there would be an escalation in drug use and related crime. Also, addition of more drugs to the pressing problems with "legal drugs" (alcohol and nicotine) would be very detrimental.
      3. It is thought that prevention efforts should target susceptible aggregates such as women, adolescents, and members of minority groups to seek to reduce the harm.
      4. Substance use patterns should be routinely assessed by nurses in all health care contexts in which client histories are performed.
   B. Treatment
      1. Several types of treatment programs exist.
         a. Treatment for substance abuse problems may be conducted on an inpatient or outpatient basis.
         b. Treatment may be either voluntary or compulsory.
         c. Treatment may be either pharmacologically based or "drug-free."
      2. Treatment is based on the severity of the problem as well as pertinent cultural factors; therefore, treatment should follow a thorough assessment.
         a. The history should include information about lifestyle, employment, relationships, and self-perception.
         b. Specific questions regarding smoking, drinking, and illicit drug use should be included.
         c. Screening tools may be incorporated into the interview and history.
         d. A physical examination should also be completed to identify pre- or co-existing problems that may impact treatment or be affected by it.
      3. Intervention often begins with providing information about the effects of alcohol and drugs. A discussion of a solution to abuse-related problems to remove barriers to intervention (such as shame, denial, guilt, fear, and erroneous preconceptions and attitudes about alcohol and drug problems) usually follows.
      4. Detoxification is short-term treatment designed to manage acute withdrawal from the substance. It involves medical intervention to reduce side effects of the substance and help stabilize the client.
      5. Other treatment programs include group therapy, individual therapy, counseling, education, 12-step groups, aversion therapy, use of Antabuse or methadone, hypnosis, occupational therapy, and psychoanalysis.

6. Several important points should be noted regarding treatment of substance abuse.
   a. Treatment should be tailored to the specific needs of the individual.
   b. Treatment should stress the importance of family intervention to engage important social network members in the process.
   c. Treatment is not recovery, but a part of the recovery process; therefore, it must address the after-care needs of the client.
   d. A comprehensive treatment approach will recognize the multifaceted nature of dependence and addiction and attempt to address these influences within the course of the treatment.
7. Evaluation of the effectiveness of therapy should include several criteria.
   a. Number of days abstinent
   b. Employability or work attendance
   c. Spouse's assessment of client's functionality
   d. Regular attendance at 12-step groups
   e. Compliance with appointments
   f. Absence of psychiatric symptoms (depression or anxiety)
   g. Self-report of progress
C. Pharmacotherapies—Several pharmacotherapeutic agents are being used successfully as adjuncts to assist in treatment of substance abuse.
   1. Disulfiram (Antabuse) has been widely used to treat people with alcohol abuse. Within minutes of alcohol consumption, disulfiram produces a severe reaction including flushing, tachycardia, nausea, headache, and chest pain.
   2. Naltrexone (Trexan, ReVia) is a long-acting narcotic antagonist used as an adjunct in treatment of opiate dependence. It works by blocking the effects of the opiate.
   3. Methadone is a long-acting oral opioid that has been used to facilitate the return of addicted people to "normal functioning." Methadone may be used as either a detoxifying agent or a maintenance drug.
   4. Buprenorphine is an opioid agonist/antagonist that is used to treat opiate-dependent people with concurrent cocaine dependence.
   5. Other pharmacotherapeutic agents, such as clonidine (Catapres), are used to reduce withdrawal symptoms of sweating, anxiety, hypertension, increased gastrointestinal motility, diarrhea, and tachycardia.

D. Issues unique to substance abuse—Dealing with substance abuse presents a number of unique issues that must be handled carefully.
   1. Encroachment on individual right of privacy
   2. Informed consent
   3. Self-determination
E. Relapse prevention
   1. Relapse prevention aims to prepare the client for the relapse situation in the hope of preventing it or minimizing its negative impact on the recovery process.
   2. In relapse prevention, cognitive reframing, role-playing, and planning for coping with negative mood states are done to prepare the client to meet the challenge of potential relapse.
F. Mutual help groups—Mutual help groups are associations that are voluntarily formed and operate through face-to-face supportive interaction that focuses on a mutual goal. They are usually organized by recovering substance abusers or individuals recovering from compulsive behavior patterns.
   1. The first mutual help group was Alcoholics Anonymous (AA).
      a. AA was founded in 1935 by a small group of white male alcoholics who found a way to stay sober one day at a time through meeting with others like themselves.
      b. The early members developed 12 steps to guide the recovery process.
      c. Alcoholics Anonymous is viewed as relatively successful.
   2. Other 12-step programs have been developed by adapting AA's approach and applying it to similar addictive problems.
      a. Narcotics Anonymous
      b. Gamblers Anonymous
      c. Overeaters Anonymous
   3. Other non-12-step mutual help groups have been developed in response to negative experiences in such groups.
      a. "Women for Sobriety" was organized to replace or augment AA for women who find AA's literature and customs inappropriate or sexist.
      b. "Secular Sobriety Groups" were organized to meet the needs of atheists, agnostics, and others who are unable to accept dependence on a "higher power" in their recovery.
      c. Other groups are available for a variety of addictive problems.

V. Social Network Involvement
  A. Family and friends—The social network of the substance abuser can be quite influential in helping the individual alter behaviors in a positive manner; alternatively, they can also aid the substance abuser in self-destruction. There is evidence that substance use and abuse often occurs in the context of social interactions.
    1. The nurse should attempt to identify important members of the individual's social network and determine how they support the client.
    2. The family has suffered the effects of the substance abuse emotionally, socially, economically, physically, and spiritually; thus, the family's problems must be acknowledged and treated.
    3. *Codependency* is a term that recognizes identifiable patterns of interaction that describe the addicted family system.
      a. These patterns or behaviors help to maintain the family in the pattern that supports substance abuse and addiction.
      b. Family treatment is essential in substance abuse because the family can be instrumental in enabling the continuation of drug abuse through protection and support of the individual.
  B. Effects on the family—Substance abuse is a family disease because it affects the entire family system with potentially adverse psychological and physical consequences for the family members as well as the abuser.
    1. A functional family system is open and flexible and allows its members to be free to be themselves. All family members are able to get their needs met in a reasonable way.
    2. A dysfunctional family is composed of closed a system with fixed, rigid roles.
      a. A major purpose of the system is to deny the substance abuse of the abuser and keep the family secret.
      b. Communication is unbalanced, and family functions are centered around the abuser's behavior.
      c. Individual needs of the other family members often go unmet.
      d. Denial is central to the functioning of the family system.
      e. Adult children of dysfunctional families often carry these roles and coping mechanisms into adult life. Many become substance abusers or spouses of substance abusers.

  C. Professional enablers—Health care professionals can also contribute to the initiation and continuation of substance abuse and dependency.
    1. One example is the overprescription of psychoactive medications by physicians.
      a. The addictive potential of analgesics and anti-anxiety medications may be ignored.
      b. Long-term goals for treatment of medical problems and non-pharmacologic management of pain and anxiety are possible alternatives.
    2. Reluctance on the part of the health care worker to suggest the possibility of addiction may also support the addiction.

VI. Vulnerable Aggregates
  A. Substance abuse problems clearly affect some populations more severely than others.
    1. *Vulnerable aggregates* are groups that are more susceptible to experience substance abuse problems, may deteriorate more quickly, or have fewer sources of support for recovery compared with the traditional comparison group of middle-class, Euro-American, heterosexual men.
    2. Race or ethnic group, age, gender, ethnic practices, religious beliefs, economic conditions, availability of options and alternatives, and physiologic susceptibility are factors that may influence the incidence and type of substance abuse.
  B. Adolescents
    1. Because adolescence is a period of transition and social stress, substances are often used for the first time during this period.
    2. Peer pressure, physiologic immaturity of the user, social role pressures, risk-taking orientation, and lack of other recreational alternatives contribute to substance abuse by adolescents.
    3. Use begins early.
      a. Reported experimentation rates by 8th grade
        1) Alcohol—70%
        2) Marijuana—10%
        3) Cocaine—2%
        4) Cigarettes—44%
      b. Reported experimentation rates by 12th grade
        1) Alcohol—88%
        2) Marijuana—37%
        3) Cocaine—8%
        4) Cigarettes—63%

4. Because cigarettes and alcohol are typically tried before illicit drugs, they are considered "gateway drugs" and are increasingly the focus of prevention efforts.
5. The younger the age for initiation of drug or alcohol use, the more likely heavy use will develop.
6. The majority of adolescent alcohol abusers also use other drugs, such as marijuana and cocaine.
7. Adolescents from poor socioeconomic groups face multiple problems, and adolescents seeking treatment present with severe complications, including learning disorders, borderline personality disorders, and physical, sexual, and emotional abuse and neglect.
8. Prevention efforts for adolescents
   a. Most prevention efforts have emphasized drug education with an abstinence philosophy ("just say no").
   b. Increasingly, drug education in schools is focusing on the choices of adolescents and the consequences associated with these choices.
   c. Deterrents to illicit drug use among adolescents include negative parent attitudes toward drug use, absence of substance-abusing role models, and existence of an extended family support system.
C. Elderly
   1. The elderly are vulnerable to substance abuse problems because of diminished physiologic tolerance, increased use of medically prescribed drugs, and the effects of cultural and social isolation.
   2. Alcohol and drug abuse constitutes 10% of all admissions to geriatric mental health facilities.
   3. The prevalence of alcohol abuse in the elderly is about the same as that of the general population.
   4. Illicit drug use is not common, but abuse of prescription drugs, particularly narcotic analgesics, sedatives, and hypnotics, is common, especially among elderly women.
   5. Health care professionals often contribute to prescription drug problems by failure to assess medication use thoroughly.
D. Women
   1. Because of social and cultural factors, non-white women, low-income or no-income women, lesbians, and working-class women

are especially at risk for substance abuse problems.
   2. Research has shown that women may be more susceptible to effects of chemicals than men.
   3. Drug-dependent women report physical and medical problems more often, and alcoholism appears to progress more rapidly in women than in men.
   4. Substance abuse during pregnancy is estimated at about 11% and produces serious concerns for the developing fetus.
      a. Cocaine is associated with increased risk of spontaneous abortion, premature delivery, and abruptio placentae.
      b. Infants exposed to cocaine in utero are hyper-irritable, subject to seizures, and at risk for SIDS as well as long-term learning disabilities, behavioral problems, mental retardation, and physical handicaps.
E. Minority groups
   1. Members of ethnic and racial minority groups are particularly susceptible to the effects of substance abuse and dependency.
      a. Poverty, oppression, underemployment, decreased job opportunities, and racism contribute to the use of a variety of substances to escape from the realities of their environment.
      b. Stress, social causation, cultural values, and role models may encourage substance use and abuse.
   2. When working with minority groups, it is important for health care professionals to recognize the sociopolitical and socioeconomic factors that affect substance use, abuse, and dependency.
      a. Recovery in minority populations may be hindered by returning to an environment in which there is pressure to use. Conflict and confusion with the family and culture may result.
      b. Health care providers must recognize that this aggregate will encounter many barriers that make treatment and long-term recovery extremely difficult.
   3. Several barriers to treating substance abuse successfully exist in minority populations.
      a. The effects of a history of racism and psychological handicaps on self-esteem and self-awareness
      b. Poverty, underemployment, and unemployment

c. Availability and accessibility of both drugs and alcohol in the community
d. Lifestyles that accept and value "hustling" over menial and low-paying jobs
e. Economic rewards that come from selling drugs
f. Inadequate social support for recovery as an alternative lifestyle
F. Other aggregates
1. Dual diagnosis
a. Because substance abuse is the most common psychopathology in the general population, there exists a group of people with one or more psychiatric diagnoses in addition to substance abuse (dual diagnosis).
b. Treatment and integration of people with dual diagnoses is often complicated by the need for the individual to take prescribed psychotropic medications.
2. HIV-positive individuals—Substance abusers are at increased risk of HIV-related health deficits for the following reasons.
a. High-risk sexual or drug practices
b. Sharing hypodermic needles
c. Impairment of the immune system through chronic substance use
d. Enhanced physical and mental deterioration following infection
e. Fewer available supportive relationships to cope with HIV diagnosis
f. Use of drugs or alcohol to cope with the distress of an HIV diagnosis
3. Health care professionals—Physicians, nurses, dentists, and pharmacists are vulnerable to substance abuse.
a. The main addictions among this group are to alcohol or narcotics.
b. Increased access to drugs, belief in pharmaceutical solutions, and work-related stress places health care professionals at increased risk.
4. Other at-risk groups
a. Low-income Hispanic males
b. Native Americans
VII. **Nursing Perspective on Substance Abuse**—In the past decade, nursing has become more involved in prevention of substance abuse and interventions. Educational coursework related to alcohol and drug abuse is now recommended for inclusion in general nursing school curricula.
A. Common nursing diagnoses for clients with substance abuse and dependency problems

1. Alteration in comfort related to withdrawal symptoms
2. Self-care deficits
3. Hopelessness related to depression over substance abuse
4. Powerlessness related to loss of control over use
5. Dysfunctional family processes
6. Alteration in nutrition (lower than body requirements)
7. Social isolation
8. Ineffective individual coping
9. Potential for violence
10. Anxiety
B. Community health nurses and substance abusers
1. Substance abuse or dependence either contributes to or complicates the course of many other illnesses and injuries.
2. Substance abuse is often a direct cause of traumatic injuries, crime, and domestic violence.
3. Ignoring substance abuse problems frequently leads to lack of progress or improvement in a health condition and the client's inability to carry out needed health practices.
C. Attitude toward substance abusers
1. Nurses have historically had ambivalent attitudes toward alcoholics and drug addicts.
2. Frequently, substance abusers are difficult clients in health care settings. They may be uncooperative, antisocial, manipulative, and demanding.
3. Nurses should convey an accepting, nonjudgmental attitude when caring for substance abusers.

VIII. **Nursing Interventions in the Community**
A. Community health nurses should provide accurate assessments, including a family history that questions personal drug and alcohol use.
B. Environmental clues in the home should also be assessed.
C. One of the primary tasks of intervention and treatment with the substance-dependent individual is to break down denial.
1. Family and significant others can assist with the process, but they may have to overcome their own denial of the problems.
2. Referral to community education programs and mutual help groups such as Alcoholics Anonymous and Narcotics Anonymous is an intervention that is often helpful to family and significant others.

D. Several traditional community health nursing roles and interventions are appropriate to use with substance abusers.
   1. Health teaching regarding addictive illness and effects of different substances
   2. Providing direct nursing care for substance abuse and dependence-related medical problems
   3. Counseling clients and families about problems related to substance abuse
   4. Collaborating with other disciplines to ensure continuity of care
   5. Coordinating health care services for the client to prevent prescription drug abuse and avoid fragmentation of care
   6. Providing consultation to non-medical professionals and lay personnel
   7. Facilitating care through appropriate referrals and followup

TEACHING STRATEGIES

1. Divide the class into groups of two or three. Have each group contact a 12-step program in the area, visit a meeting, and report impressions to the class.
2. Encourage students to collect data on illegal substance abuse in the community. What aggregates appear to be most affected? What community resources are available for treatment of addictions?
3. Divide the class into two groups. Have them examine the issues surrounding legalization or decriminalization of currently illegal drugs. During class, select representatives from each group and have them debate the issues.

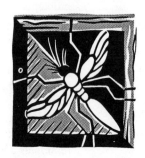

CHAPTER
24

Communicable Disease

ANNOTATED LEARNING OBJECTIVES

1. *Discuss the routes of transmission of infection.*

    Direct transmission refers to the immediate transfer of an infectious agent from an infected host or reservoir to an appropriate portal of entry in the human host through physical contact or droplets in the air. *Indirect transmission* is the spread of infection through vehicles such as inanimate objects (fomites) and arthropods (mosquitoes and ticks). *Airborne transmission* involves suspensions, particles of dust, aerosols, and droplet nuclei which are inhaled by the individual, causing disease.

2. *Identify the protocols for notifiable diseases within the Centers for Disease Control Monitoring and Surveillance System.*

    The CDC has a list of all diseases that must be reported on a weekly basis or on a monthly basis, as well as those that should be reported when encountered. Community health nurses are part of the team responsible for identification and surveillance of outbreaks of communicable disease for containment and monitoring purposes. A possible case of a notifiable disease is reported to the local health department for confirmation. All health care workers providing primary care are responsible for reporting notifiable diseases.

3. *List three communicable diseases that are currently causing high morbidity in the United States, and identify the epidemiological indicators of racial-ethnic disparity.*

    Hepatitis B is becoming increasingly common in the United States. Hepatitis B is spread through blood products, sexual activity, and sharing contaminated needles. Infection can cause severe disease and even death, but many people are asymptomatic. Some people develop chronic hepatitis and become carriers. Carrier status is associated with primary hepatic carcinoma. Hepatitis B is preventable by vaccine, which should be available to people at high risk, including homosexual men, IV drug users, and children born to Asian-American women.

    The incidence of pulmonary tuberculosis has increased dramatically in some U.S. aggregates in the last several years. African-Americans between the ages of 25 and 44 have the highest rates, followed by older whites. Drug-resistant strains, particularly in HIV-positive individuals, are becoming increasingly more common.

    AIDS and HIV infection rates are becoming more common among African-Americans and Hispanics, largely due to IV drug use and unsafe sexual practices. Although more white males have contracted the disease, increasing prevalence among women and their offspring have been recognized.

4. *Specify which immunizations are required by law in the United States, for what ages, and discuss their efficacy.*

    Diphtheria/tetanus/pertussis (DPT) is required at 2, 4, 6 months with boosters at 15–18 months and 4–6 years. Polio vaccine is required at 2, 4, 12–15 months, and 4–6 years. Measles/mumps/rubella vaccine is required at 15 months and 4–5 or 11–12 years.

    In addition to the required immunizations, other immunizations are recommended for at-risk children. *Haemophilus influenza* B is given at 2, 4, 6, and 15 months; hepatitis B may be given at birth, 2 months, and 6 months.

    Each of these vaccines has approximately a 95% success rate, particularly if the schedule is followed correctly. Complications are rare.

5. *Discuss the prevalence and risk factors involved in the acquisition of AIDS and other sexually transmitted diseases and identify methods for control.*

Chlamydial and gonorrheal infections are common. Although frequently causing no symptoms, both illnesses can cause pelvic inflammatory disease in women and obstructive infertility. Screening should be performed yearly. Treatment is easy and inexpensive; however, emphasis should focus on prevention through abstinence and "safer sex."

Herpes simplex virus is becoming more prevalent. Although not life-threatening except to the neonate during delivery, it can be very painful and debilitating. The spread of herpes can be prevented by abstinence from sexual activity during outbreaks and use of condoms.

AIDS/HIV infections are ultimately fatal. Control is through education, provision of easy access to condoms and clean needles for IV drug use, and pregnancy prevention. Secondary prevention efforts include early diagnosis, counseling, and treatment to increase the interval between infection and onset of the illness. Universal precautions by all health care workers and thorough screening of blood products are also employed to limit infection.

6. *Explain the difference among prevention, control, elimination, and eradication of communicable diseases.*

Prevention of a communicable disease refers to reducing or eliminating exposure or susceptibility to a disease. *Control* of a communicable disease is the reduction of incidence or prevalence of a given disease at any point in time. *Elimination* of a communicable disease involves controlling it within a specified geographical area such as a single country, an island, or a continent and reducing the prevalence and incidence to eventual eradication. *Eradication* refers to reducing the incidence of a disease worldwide to zero as a function of deliberate efforts with no need for further control measures.

LECTURE OUTLINE

Community health nurses participate in health promotion and disease prevention interventions and programs related to the prevention and control of communicable diseases within the community. This is accomplished through employment of a multidisciplinary team composed of sanitary engineering, public health, nursing and medicine. Most people who contract communicable diseases are cared for at home and are seen on an outpatient basis. Community health nurses play an important role

in the continuity of care for these people, as well as in disease prevention and control.

I. **The Communicable Disease Spectrum**
   A. During the last three decades, many efforts have been taken, and goals written, addressing reduction of communicable diseases throughout the world.
   B. Enhancing immunization against vaccine-preventable diseases, in both children and adults, is one of the keys to meeting these goals.
   C. Application of community-based health programs can assist by interrupting or preventing transmission and by providing an assessment of the risk factors that impede health and increase the likelihood of transmission.
   D. Identified risk factors include environmental, socioeconomic, political, education, employment, and health factors.

II. **Transmission**
   A. Direct transmission
      1. Direct transmission implies the immediate transfer of an infectious agent from an infected host or reservoir to an appropriate portal of entry in the human host through physical contact or droplets in the air.
      2. Examples of diseases resulting from direct transmission are scabies, herpes, mononucleosis, gonorrhea, and chicken pox.
   B. Indirect transmission—Indirect transmission is the spread of infection through vehicles such as inanimate objects (fomites), animals, and arthropods (vectors such as mosquitoes and ticks).
      1. Indirect transmission can occur in the form of contaminated food or water, blood products, or human transplants.
      2. Types of indirect transmission
         a. Contaminated fomites can be any inanimate object, material, or substance that acts as a transport agent for the pathogen, introducing it to a suitable port of entry in the human host. Fomites include toothbrushes, dressings, cooking or eating utensils, currency, books, and telephones.
         b. Mechanical vector transmission does not involve multiplication or growth of the microbe within the vector itself. The microbe is transported when the vector mechanically carries the agent in its intestinal tract, on its feet, or by flying over or crawling on the human host or the human's food supply.

c. Biological transmission occurs when the parasite grows or multiplies inside the vector or arthropod through extrinsic incubation. This typically occurs in contaminated food or water or in the intestinal tract or the circulatory system of the nonvertebrate host and must occur for the parasite to infect a person.

d. The mode of transmission from the vector to the human host is often a bite, a sting, or the deposit of fecal material on the skin at, or near, a puncture wound, or ingestion of the contaminated water or food.

3. Examples of diseases that occur through indirect transmission include tetanus, rabies, botulism, plague, and malaria.

C. Fecal-oral transmission can be both direct and indirect.

1. It can occur through the ingestion of water or food that has been fecally contaminated, or through engagement in oral-genital sexual activity.

2. Examples of diseases that may be transmitted through this route are giardiasis, hepatitis A, cholera, and typhoid fever.

D. Airborne transmission

1. Airborne transmission involves suspensions, particles of dust, aerosols and droplet nuclei.

2. The timeframe in which an airborne particle can remain suspended greatly influences its virility and infectivity. The smaller the particle, the less likely it is to settle out of the air too quickly, and the greater the chance of infecting the human host.

3. Droplet nuclei are small particles that separate from droplets through evaporation of water or fluid.

a. Once this separation occurs, they can fall on the floor until they are kicked up as dust and inhaled into the lungs.

b. If droplet nuclei are inhaled with the fluid still attached, they may separate in the respiratory tree and be inhaled into the alveolar space.

c. The mode of transmission for tuberculosis is droplet nuclei from airborne infections.

4. Examples of airborne-transmitted diseases are mumps, common cold, pertussis, measles, and tuberculosis.

E. Transmission can also be vertical, horizontal, transplacental, or across a group of people, such as within a family.

1. For transmission, there must be a human portal of entry (host) and a microbe from a source or reservoir (agent).

2. Environmental factors, such as crowding, pollution, and nutritional status, may also influence the transmission of communicable diseases.

III. **Immunity**

A. *Immunity* refers to protection from infection.

1. The concept of *herd immunity* states that those not immunized will be safe if at least 80% of the population has been vaccinated.

2. *Natural immunity* is an innate resistance to a specific antigen or toxin.

3. *Acquired immunity* is derived from actual exposure to the specific infectious agent, toxin, or vaccine.

4. *Active immunity* is present when the body can build its own antibodies that provide protection against a bacterial or other antigenic substance.

5. *Passive immunity* is temporary resistance that has been donated to the host through the transfusion of plasma proteins, immunoglobulins, or antitoxins or from mother to neonate transplacentally. Passive immunity lasts only as long as these substances remain in the bloodstream.

B. Vaccine failure

1. Primary vaccine failure is the failure of a vaccine to contribute any level of immunogenicity. This may be the result of improper care of the vaccines, rendering them ineffective, or the result of an individual's failure to seroconvert following exposure to the vaccine.

2. Secondary vaccine failure is the waning of immunogenicity after eliciting an initial immune response.

IV. **Prevention**—Prevention of communicable disease should be carried out at the primary, secondary, and tertiary levels. Examples of primary prevention interventions are teaching good handwashing and toileting to prevent fecal-oral contamination and good general personal and household hygiene to protect against vectors (rats, roaches) and food contamination. Environmental sanitation and "safer sex" practices are other examples of primary prevention.

V. **Universal Blood and Body Fluid Precautions**

A. Universal blood and body fluid precautions are recommended by the Centers for Disease Control (CDC).

B. The precautions assume that all patients are infectious for HIV and other blood-borne pathogens; therefore all body fluids should be considered infectious.

C. These precautions should be used by all health care personnel in every setting that includes provision of care.

VI. Defining and Reporting Cases

A. The CDC has developed a list of all diseases that must be reported to the CDC on a weekly basis, those that should be reported on a monthly basis, and those that must be reported when encountered.

B. The CDC monitors national trends in reported communicable diseases.

C. Reports for the entire nation and for individual geographic regions and states are published each week in the *Morbidity and Mortality Weekly Report (MMWR)*.

D. The community health nurse has a vital role in prevention, case finding, reporting, and control of communicable diseases.

VII. Control—Control of a communicable disease is the reduction of incidence or prevalence of a given disease at any point in time.

VIII. Elimination

A. The process of eliminating a communicable disease involves controlling it within a specified geographical area such as a country, island, or continent, and reducing the prevalence and incidence to eventual eradication.

B. Diseases that have been targeted for elimination by the year 2000 include polio, leprosy, and measles.

IX. Eradication

A. *Eradication* refers to reducing the incidence of a disease worldwide to zero as a function of deliberate efforts, with no need for further control measures. Smallpox was declared "eradicated" in 1977.

B. Factors that contribute to the feasibility of eradication include the following.
1. Human host only
2. Easy diagnosis (obvious clinical manifestations)
3. Limited duration
4. Limitied intensity of infection
5. Lifelong immunity after infection
6. Highly seasonal transmission
7. Availability of a vaccine

C. A number of other diseases have been targeted for eventual global eradication. These include rubella, polio, and mumps.

X. Vaccine-Preventable Diseases

A. Recommended vaccine schedules
1. The American Academy of Pediatrics, the American Academy of Family Physicians, and the Advisory Committee on Immunization Practices have developed a schedule for childhood vaccinations.
   a. According to the schedule, by the age of 18 months, each child should have four doses of DTP vaccine, three doses of oral or injected polio vaccine, three to four doses of Hib conjugate, three doses of hepatitis B, and one dose of measles/mumps/rubella vaccine.
   b. The schedule is quite complex, and compliance with routine vaccination schedules remains one of the greatest hindrances for global immunization programs.
2. Vaccines to prevent varicella and hepatitis A are available and may be recommended for some children.

B. Vaccines
1. Vaccines are either live and inactivated or killed (inactivated), thus leaving only the antigenic property necessary to stimulate the human immune system to produce antibodies.
   a. Examples of live attenuated vaccines include MMR, polio, varicella, and BCG.
   b. Inactivated vaccines include rabies, pertussis, cholera, hepatitis A and hepatitis B.
2. Vaccines can be prepared in several ways. They may be suspended in solution, protected with preservatives, stabilizers, or antibiotics, or they may be mixed with adjuvants.

C. Types of immunization
1. Vaccination is the administration of a vaccine or toxoid that confers active immunity by stimulating the body to produce antibodies or antitoxins.
2. Immunization includes not only vaccines for active immunity, but also passive immunogenic solutions such as immune globulins and antitoxins.

D. Vaccine storage, transport, and handling
1. Vaccines should be safely stored, transported, and handled at all times.
2. Improper storage allows the vaccines to be exposed to high temperatures, which can cause them to lose their potency and render them useless.

3. Vaccine failure can frequently be traced to improper vaccine storage.
E. Vaccine administration and routes
   1. Vaccines are designed with specific types of administration needs.
   2. If routes and procedures are not adhered to, vaccine efficacy may be adversely affected.
   3. Attention to sterile technique, ensuring that the needle is not in a blood vessel, and careful choice of needle for proper administration (intramuscular, subcutaneous) and size of the patient are important.
F. Vaccine dosages—The specified dosage of each vaccine is indicated in the package insert and should be strictly adhered to.
G. Vaccine spacing
   1. To avoid age-related complications or interference with the immune response, all children should be immunized according the recommended schedule.
   2. Clinically stable premature infants should adhere to the same schedule as term infants.
   3. Many vaccines can be administered simultaneously without contraindication.
H. Vaccine hypersensitivity
   1. Occasionally, individuals experience adverse effects, such as allergic reactions ranging from local inflammation to severe systemic responses.
   2. Reactions may be due to vaccine components (eggs, egg proteins, antibiotics, or preservatives).
   3. Fever is not a contraindication for vaccination if the risk of infection is high or if the chance for revaccination is unreliable.
   4. Pregnancy is not a contraindication for immunization for most vaccines; however, MMR should be avoided whenever possible.
   5. Immunocompromised patients should not receive live vaccines such as the oral polio vaccine.
I. Vaccine documentation
   1. Legal documentation of vaccinations is important for both the individual and the provider for future administration and for followup of hypersensitivity reactions.
   2. Both individual and provider immunization records should be carefully maintained.
   3. For each patient, the health care provider is responsible for maintaining records that include the patient's name, date immunized, vaccine type, vaccine manufacturer, vaccine lot number, and the name, title, and address of the person administering the vaccine.

J. Reporting adverse events and vaccine related injuries—Health care providers must report specific post-vaccination adverse events to the Vaccine Adverse Events Reporting System, which has a 24-hour recorded telephone message system.

XI. **Vaccine Needs for Special Groups**
A. Adolescents and young adults
   1. Following the 1989-1991 measles epidemic in the United States, it was determined that all children should receive a second MMR.
   2. It is also important that children receive the recommended 10-year dose of tetanus and diphtheria toxoids (Td).
   3. In 1995, the ACIP recommended an adolescent schedule, adding a hepatitis B series and the varicella vaccine for youths who have no history of chicken pox.
   4. Many colleges and university require proof of immunizations before enrollment.
B. Adults and elders
   1. Vaccine-preventable diseases continue to cause deaths in adults, most often affecting elderly populations.
   2. In 1994, new recommendations for adult vaccinations were developed.
      a. Assess the current immunization status of all adults.
      b. Administer Td toxoids if indicated.
      c. Determine whether the adult has risk factors that suggest the need for pneumococcal and influenza vaccinations.
C. Immunosuppression
   1. Altered or compromised immune status may be due to HIV infection, leukemia, lymphoma, congenial immunodeficiency, radiation, large doses of corticosteroids, or other factors.
   2. If the individual is severely immunosuppressed, live virus or bacteria vaccines could pose a serious threat to health.
   3. Killed or inactivated vaccines are not problematic and can follow the same recommended administration schedule.
D. Pregnancy
   1. The Td vaccine is the only vaccine routinely indicated for susceptible pregnant women.
   2. Hepatitis B, influenza, and pneumococcal vaccines are recommended for at-risk pregnant women.
   3. MMR vaccine is contraindicated when pregnancy is known.
   4. Live virus vaccines (OPV and yellow fever) are not recommended during pregnancy.

XII. Vaccine-Preventable Diseases
A. Diphtheria
1. Diphtheria is an acute bacterial disease most commonly affecting the upper respiratory tract (nose, tonsils, larynx, and pharynx).
2. Complications may result, including severe swelling of the neck, thrombocytopenia, neuritis, and myocarditis.
3. The case fatality rate is 10-15%.
4. It is transmitted through direct contact with an infected individual and has an incubation period of 2–5 days.
5. Diphtheria is rare in the United States, but it continues to be a major cause of morbidity and mortality in young children worldwide.
6. Diphtheria-tetanus-pertussis is a triple-antigen vaccine that combines diphtheria and tetanus toxoids with the pertussis vaccine.
   a. It is recommended as a series for children under the age of seven.
   b. The primary childhood series is given in five successive doses at 2, 4, 6, 18 months and 4–5 years.
   c. Boosters, usually combining diphtheria and tetanus toxoids, are given every ten years.
7. Diphtheria toxoid may cause soreness at the injection site and fever. Antibody formation lasts about 10 years.
B. *Haemophilus Influenza* type B (Hib)
1. Hib is an acute invasive bacterial infection usually affecting children younger than 5 years, and should not be confused with influenza types A, B and C, which are viral diseases.
2. Hib-associated illnesses include meningitis, epiglottitis, otitis media, pneumonia, and arthritis.
3. Worldwide, Hib is the major cause of bacterial meningitis in children younger than 5 years.
4. Hib is transmitted by droplets from nasal and oral secretions.
5. The incubation period is short (2–4 days).
6. Vaccination against Hib may be given as a monovalent vaccine (only Hib) or in a DTP-Hib combination.
C. Hepatitis A and B—Although there are several forms of viral hepatitis, vaccines are only available for hepatitis A and B.
1. Hepatitis A (HAV)
   a. HAV is an acute viral infection that presents with fever, anorexia, and general malaise, followed by jaundice which may last two weeks.
   b. It is transmitted through fecal-oral contamination of food and water and has an incubation period of 15–50 days.
   c. HAV is endemic in many developing countries.
   d. In the United States there are periodic outbreaks, often in child care centers and schools, and hepatitis A is fairly common.
   e. With the introduction of the new vaccine, it is expected that the incidence of HAV will decline over the next decade.
   f. The vaccine is given in a two-dose series and is recommended for people engaged in "high risk" activities (those traveling to a country of high endemicity, communities experiencing an outbreak, people with chronic liver disease, American Indian or Alaskan natives, laboratory workers, handlers of primate animals, staff of child day care centers, and males having sex with other males).
   g. Soreness at the site of injection is the only common side effect.
2. Hepatitis B (HBV) (serum hepatitis)
   a. HBV is a viral infection that ranges from asymptomatic illness to generalized nonspecific symptoms (anorexia, nausea, vomiting) followed by jaundice. It occasionally results in fulminant fatal hepatitis.
   b. It is transmitted through direct contact with contaminated blood and body secretions, transplacentally, and through sexual intercourse.
   c. HBV is endemic worldwide and has an incubation period of 45 days to 6 months.
   d. The carrier status of chronic disease is extremely dangerous because severe damage to the liver and liver cancer may result.
   e. Eighty percent of all cases of primary liver cancer are due to HBV.
   f. HBV vaccination became part of the routine childhood immunization schedule in the early 1990s.
      1) The vaccine is in a three-dose series.
      2) In addition to infants, vaccine administration is recommended for all pregnant women who are seropositive for HBsAg (which indicates a

carrier status), their infants, all children born to Asian-American mothers, health care workers, high-risk groups such as homosexual men, and individuals who work in institutions for the developmentally disabled.

  g. Although there is an effective vaccine for prevention of hepatitis B, eradication of the disease is problematic for several reasons.

    1) the vaccine is very expensive and thus can be prohibitive for those at highest risk of contracting the disease.

    2) The presence of carrier status (as many as 300 million people worldwide are infected) prevents eradication.

    3) For universal eradication, there must be immunization of infants and adolescents worldwide.

    4) Noncompliance with the second and third inoculations can inhibit the success of seroconversion.

D. Influenza types A, B, and C

  1. Influenza is an acute viral respiratory infection that may be confused with the common cold or other common respiratory illness.

  2. Influenza has three types.

    a. A (responsible for most epidemics)

    b. B (responsible for regional outbreaks)

    c. C (less common; usually results in mild illness)

  3. Symptoms of influenza include cough, fever, headache, myalgia, sore throat, and malaise.

  4. Complications include pneumonia, otitis media, meningitis and Reye's syndrome.

  5. The peak transmission season for influenza in the United States runs from November through February.

  6. Groups at greatest risk for complications from influenza include the elderly, individuals with underlying health problems, health care workers, and others in close contact with individuals at high risk.

  7. Influenza vaccine should be encouraged for patients at risk.

  8. Individuals should be revaccination with the most current vaccine every fall.

E. Measles

  1. Measles is an acute viral infection that presents with fever, cough, conjunctivitis, Koplik's spots, and a red rash that begins on the face and becomes generalized.

  2. Complications include pneumonia, diarrhea, encephalitis, and death.

  3. It is highly infectious and is transmitted through droplets and indirect contact with nasal secretions of an infected person.

  4. There are 45 million cases of measles yearly, resulting in approximately 1.1 million deaths in infants and children.

  5. Measles vaccination is a two-dose series, with doses administered between 15 months and 4–5 years.

    a. Measles-mumps-rubella (MMR) is a combined live attenuated vaccine.

    b. It is contraindicated for pregnant women, immunosuppressed people, and those sensitive to neomycin or eggs.

    c. The vaccine may cause malaise and fever for as long as 12 days after inoculation.

F. Mumps

  1. Mumps is an acute systemic viral disease that presents with fever and painful swelling of the salivary and parotid glands.

  2. Complications include meningitis, encephalitis, permanent hearing impairment, and orchitis.

  3. Mumps is transmitted through droplets and direct contact with saliva of infected individuals.

  4. Mumps vaccines are usually given in combination with measles and rubella vaccines in the MMR.

G. Pertussis

  1. Pertussis, or whooping cough, is an acute bacterial infection that begins with an upper respiratory cough and proceeds into a paroxysmal stage of coughing ending in vomiting.

  2. Complications include seizure, pneumonia, encephalopathy, and death.

  3. It is transmitted by direct contact with respiratory secretions of an infected individual and has an incubation period of 7–10 days.

  4. Most cases of pertussis are in children less than four years old.

  5. The pertussis vaccine is usually combined with tetanus and diphtheria toxoids (DTP), and more recently with Hib also.

  6. Vaccine is recommended for children from 2 months to 6 years.

  7. Complications from the vaccine increase with age.

8. Reactions from the vaccine may include neurological symptoms, which should be reported immediately.

H. Polio
 1. Poliomyelitis is an acute enterovirus that occurs in three different types.
 2. Symptoms range from unapparent illness to severe paralysis or death.
 3. It is transmitted through airborne droplets and fecal-oral contamination and has an incubation period ranging from 7–21 days.
 4. Cases in the United States are very rare, and cases worldwide are declining.
 5. Those at risk for contracting polio are people who are not vaccinated and those who are immunosuppressed.
 6. Polio vaccines are prepared using both live and killed virus.
    a. The trivalent live attenuated virus vaccine is administered orally to children under the age of 18. The vaccine colonizes inside the body, then enters the bloodstream to stimulate an antibody response. Anyone recently immunized may excrete live attenuated virus or reverted wild-type virus in their stool.
    b. Injectible polio vaccine (IPV) contains inactivated virus and is used in many parts of the world.
 7. In 1996, the CDC recommend a change in the polio vaccination schedule to reduce the number of vaccine-related paralytic cases of polio through use of IPV for the first two doses followed by two doses of OPV. This will require an increase in the number of injections infants will need. Contraindications are immunosuppression or diarrhea and acute gastritis.

I. Rubella
 1. Rubella is a mild viral disease that presents with a maculopapular rash.
 2. Children are relatively asymptomatic, but adults may experience fever, headache, and malaise.
 3. Complications include encephalitis and thrombocytopenia.
 4. Probably the most serious complication in adults results from infection during pregnancy. In-utero rubella exposure may result in congenital defects in the fetus.
 5. Vaccination is usually given in the trivalent MMR.
 6. Contraindications include pregnancy and anaphylactic reaction to neomycin or eggs.

J. Tetanus
 1. Tetanus (lockjaw) is an acute neurological illness caused by an anaerobic bacterium that produces an exotoxin in the portal of entry.
 2. Tetanus presents with gradually worsening neurological symptoms, including painful muscle contractions and spasms. Death may result.
 3. Tetanus is transmitted indirectly through contamination of a wound with tetanus spores, which are typically found in soil contaminated by animal excretions.
 4. The incubation period is 1–20 days.
 5. Although nonexistent in the United States, neonatal tetanus is responsible for a large percentage of infant mortality in the developing world due to use of contaminated razor blades for cutting the umbilical cord after birth.
 6. Immunization usually is provided in combination with diphtheria and pertussis for infants and small children in a four-dose series.
 7. After the age of six, a child should be given the adult tetanus toxoid combined with a less potent dose of diphtheria toxoid. A booster is given every 10 years.
 8. The vaccine may cause redness and swelling at the injection site and occasionally fever.

K. Varicella (Chickenpox)
 1. Varicella is a highly contagious viral disease with variable onset.
 2. It usually produces a mild fever and malaise followed by a progressive rash which progresses from maculopapular to vesicular, then forms a crust or scab.
 3. The lesions tend to be very pruritic, and secondary bacterial infection related to scratching is the most common side effect.
 4. Transmission is by droplet infection from respiratory tract secretions, direct contact with vesicular fluid, or maternal infection during pregnancy.
 5. Latent acute re-infection can occur, usually in adulthood as shingles.
 6. Incubation ranges between 10 and 21 days after exposure.
 7. There are between 150,000 and 200,000 cases per year in the United States; 90% occur in children younger than 15 years.
 8. Susceptible adults usually have a more severe disease course and a higher case

fatality rate, accounting for 50% of deaths from varicella each year.

9. The varicella vaccine was approved and licensed by the FDA in 1995 and is now available in the United States for vaccination in children 12–18 months of age, for children 2–12, and for susceptible people who are at risk for exposure.

    a. Side effects of the vaccine include pain, soreness, redness, and swelling at the injection site.

    b. The vaccine is contraindicated for people with severe allergic reactions to neomycin and for those who are pregnant, have moderate to severe illness, or are immunocompromised.

XIII. Vaccines for International Travel—Vaccination is often recommended for individuals traveling outside of the United States into regions endemic for specific infectious disease.

A. Cholera

1. Cholera is an acute enteric bacterial infection that can cause profuse watery diarrhea, vomiting, and dehydration.

2. Complications include severe dehydration, circulatory collapse, convulsions, coma, and death.

3. Transmission of cholera is through the fecal-oral route (usually ingested) or through fecally contaminated water or food. It has an incubation period of a few hours to 5 days.

4. Cholera is very rare in the United States, but in 1992 an outbreak of 105 cases occurred.

5. The cholera vaccine is available worldwide and may be used in highly endemic areas. It provides 3–6 months of protection for 50% of individuals vaccinated.

B. Japanese encephalitis (JE)

1. Japanese encephalitis is an acute inflammatory virus.

2. It may be asymptomatic or can present with fever, headache, and disruptions to the central nervous system.

3. Complications may include hepatitis, convulsions, paralysis, and death.

4. JE is transmitted by infected mosquitoes and has an incubation period of 5–15 days.

5. Endemic areas for JE include China, Korea, Japan, Southeast Asia, India, and parts of Oceania. It is very rare in the United States.

6. The JE vaccine is an inactivated virus.

C. Meningococcus

1. Meningococcal meningitis is an acute bacterial infection that may be asymptomatic or may present with fever, headache, stiff neck, nausea and vomiting, and possibly a maculopapular or petechial rash.

2. Complications include shock, coma, and death.

3. Transmission is through airborne droplets or direct contact with an infected individual or carrier, and incubation is 2–10 days.

4. There are 3000–4000 cases each year in the United States, and meningococcal meningitis is the second most common cause of bacterial meningitis

5. Children younger than 5 years are at greatest risk for meningococcal meningitis.

6. The meningococcal vaccine is recommended for individuals entering high-risk areas and areas with epidemic outbreaks.

D. Plague

1. Plague is a serious zoonotic bacterial infection that may be asymptomatic or present with fever and painful, swollen lymph nodes.

2. Complications of plague include dissemination throughout the body.

3. Secondary pharyngeal and pneumonic plague may produce direct human transmission and has a case fatality rate of 50%.

4. Transmission of bubonic plague is through the bite of an infected flea or through direct contamination with a the infected drainage of a purulent bubo.

5. Airborne droplets from an infected individual may be responsible for transmission of pharyngeal or pneumonic plague.

6. The incubation is 2–6 days.

7. During 1993, the United States reported 10 cases of plague with one fatality.

8. The vaccine is an inactivated whole-cell bacterial preparation that is fairly effective.

E. Rabies

1. Rabies is a zoonotic viral disease that presents with progressive central nervous system involvement, including anxiety, dysphagia, and convulsions.

2. The most common complication of rabies is death.

3. Rabies is directly transmitted through the bite of an infected animal to a human host with an incubation period ranging from a few days to more than one year.

4. In the developing world, cases of rabies from dogs have become common.

5. In the United States, increasing numbers of cases have been seen in raccoons and bats.

6. When an individual is bitten by an infected animal, immediate passive immunization should be administered using rabies immune globulin. The individual should also receive active immunization with either human diploid-cell vaccine or rabies vaccine absorbed.
7. Rabies vaccine schedules are specific for pre-exposure and post-exposure prophylaxis. Pain and swelling at the site of injection are common side effects.

F. Tuberculosis (TB)
1. Tuberculosis is a mycobacterial infection that causes tubercular lesions in the lung or other organs.
2. These lesions may remain dormant for life or become reactivated at any time and progress to active pulmonary tuberculosis.
3. TB presents with early symptoms of fatigue, fever, and weight loss advancing to cough, chest pain, hemoptysis and hoarseness.
4. Mortality is high in untreated cases.
5. TB is transmitted through airborne droplets or a spray from infected individuals and has an incubation period of 2–12 weeks.
6. Those at risk for contracting TB in the United States include low socioeconomic groups living in crowded urban poverty, the homeless, immunocompromised patients, and foreign-born and minority women.
7. The Mantoux test (purified protein derivative, or PPD) is the test of choice for TB.
8. Previous vaccination with BCG is not a contraindication for administering PPD.
9. Diagnosis is made using radiography and sputum culture.
10. If a person becomes infected, a multi-drug regimen, usually combining two or three of the drugs isoniazid, rifampin, pyrazinamide, and/or ethambutol over a period of nine months is necessary.
11. The BCG vaccine is a live, attenuated bacteria that is used for prevention of TB in people who are at risk for repeated exposure and for individuals in whom other forms of preventive therapy are contraindicated. The efficacy of BCG is debated, and it is contraindicated in immunodeficient people.

G. Typhoid
1. Typhoid is a severe systemic bacterial infection that may be asymptomatic or may produce fever, headache, malaise, constipation, anorexia, rash, and lymphadenopathy.
2. Complications include "Peyer's patches" in the ilium, which can lead to perforation, hemorrhage, and adhesions of the small intestine; mental dullness; and death.
3. Typhoid is transmitted through ingestion of food or water contaminated with the urine or feces of a carrier or infected individual.
4. Typhoid is fairly rare in the United States, and the majority of cases occur in people who recently traveled outside the United States. Two vaccines are available against typhoid, and both have uncertain efficacy rates ranging between 46–96%.
5. The oral, live bacteria vaccine is contraindicated in children younger than six years and in immunocompromised patients.

H. Yellow fever
1. Yellow fever is an acute infectious arbovirus that may present with sudden onset, fever, chills, nausea, vomiting, jaundice, and hemorrhagic disorders.
2. Complications include hepatitis, coma, and death.
3. Transmission is through the bite of an infected mosquito.
4. Yellow fever has an incubation period of 3–6 days.
5. Africa and South America are the only two areas of the world in which yellow fever currently occurs.
6. The yellow fever vaccine is a live attenuated virus vaccine.
   a. It is 100% effective and provides protection for about 10 years.
   b. Contraindications to the vaccine include pregnancy and hypersensitivity to eggs or egg products. Children less than 9 months of age are also contraindicated.
   c. Slight fever, headache, and muscle pain are side effects of the vaccine.

XIV. **Sexually Transmitted Diseases**
A. Statistics
1. Sexually transmitted diseases are transferred from host to recipient through sexual intercourse and/or sexual activity and are becoming an increasing problem in the United States as well as internationally.
2. More than 50 organisms and syndromes are known to be sexually transmitted, and an estimated 12 million cases of STDs occur each year in the United States. The most common are chlamydia (4 million cases); trichomonas (3 million cases); gonorrhea (1.1 million cases); human papillomavirus

(1 million cases); herpes (500,000 cases); hepatitis B (200,000 cases); syphilis (120,000 cases) and HIV (40,000 cases).

3. STDs are not easily cured, and they may cause serious, irreversible consequences.

4. More than 20% of Americans are infected, including men and women of all ages, racial and ethnic backgrounds, and income levels.

5. Adolescents, young adults, women, minorities, and the poor have disproportionately high numbers of STDs.

6. Complications from STDs tend to occur more frequently and are more severe in women than in men.

B. AIDS/HIV

1. AIDS/HIV is caused by human immunodeficiency virus and was first recognized in 1981. It has since become a leading cause of worldwide morbidity and mortality.

2. HIV is transmitted by the following means.

   a. Sexual contact involving exchange of body fluids with an infected individual

   b. Blood transfusion or exposure to blood, blood products, or tissues of an infected person

   c. Perinatal transmission from an infected mother during pregnancy, delivery, or breast-feeding

   d. Sharing needles or syringes with an infected individual

3. An estimated 18 million adults and 1.5 million children worldwide are infected with HIV.

4. In the United States, more than 500,000 cases of AIDS have been reported to the CDC.

   a. Recently there has been a proportionate decrease among cases among whites from 60% to 43%, and a corresponding proportionate increase among blacks to 38% and Hispanics to 18%.

   b. Cases among drug users is now about 27%, and heterosexual transmission has risen to 10%, while homosexual transmission has dropped from 64% to 45%.

5. The following groups are at risk for AIDS.

   a. Adolescents, young adults, and others with multiple sexual partners

   b. Intravenous drug users and their sexual partners

   c. Gay men and their partners (both male and female)

   d. Women whose partners engage in high-risk behaviors

   e. People who engage in high-risk sexual practices (anal intercourse, prostitution, etc.).

6. A diagnosis of AIDS is based on confirmation that the individual is HIV+ and has one of the defined opportunistic conditions identified by the CDC (PCP, Kaposi's Sarcoma, TB, severe immunosuppression, invasive cervical cancer).

7, Treatment for HIV/AIDS is complex. The most commonly used medication is Zidovudine (AZT, ZDV). ZDV has recently been recommended for use to reduce perinatal transmission from infected women to their infants. Other antiviral medications and medications that prevent, treat, or manage symptoms are also used.

C. Chlamydia

1. Chlamydia is a bacterial infection and is currently the most prevalent of the STDs.

2. Chlamydial infections are often asymptomatic and can lead to ocular, pulmonary, enteric, and genital tract infections.

3. Complications of chlamydial infections include nongonococcal urethritis and epididymitis in men and obstructive infertility, ectopic pregnancy, and one-third of all cases of pelvic inflammatory disease in women.

4. Routine annual screening should be done on all sexually active patients.

5. Populations at high risk include sexually active adolescent females, women with multiple sexual partners, and African-Americans.

6. Treatment is easy, painless, and affordable.

7. As with all STDs, prevention through healthy sexual behaviors should be stressed.

D. Gonorrhea

1. Gonorrhea is a common bacterial disease.

2. In men, the infection may be asymptomatic or may present with a purulent discharge and dysuria.

3. In women, the infection is often asymptomatic or causes mild cervicitis or urethritis.

4. Complications in untreated women include endometritis, PID, salpingitis and ectopic pregnancy or infertility.

5. The incubation period is 2–7 days.

6. Some populations, especially urban African-Americans, have a very high prevalence.

7. Gonorrhea is treated by penicillin, but the organism has mutated and adapted to the point that higher doses are required, and resistant strains have developed.

8. A followup with a second drug administered orally is recommended to protect the person from underlying chlamydial infection and to prevent other resistant strains of gonorrhea.

E. Herpes simplex virus 2
1. Herpes simplex virus (HSV) is a chronic ulcerative disease that may present as small vesicles that progress to shallow, extremely painful ulcers.
2. After primary lesions disappear, the virus remains in a latent form, and a secondary episode may appear at any time.
3. Complications of HSV-2 include meningitis, encephalitis, coma, and death.
4. Because it is an ulcerative disease, the presence of ulcerative lesions places the individual at greater risk of infection with HIV.
5. In pregnant women, HSV-2 may result in neonatal HSV infection, which has a high mortality rate.
6. HSV-2 has an incubation of 3–21 days.
7. There are approximately 700,000 new cases annually in the United States.
8. Treatment may decrease the duration and symptoms in primary outbreaks and reduce the frequency and severity of recurrences. However there is no cure; therefore, emphasis should be placed on prevention.

F. Human papillomavirus
1. There are numerous types of human papillomavirus (HPV), including genital warts (condyloma).
2. There is a strong association between the presence of genital warts and the development of histological changes in genital tissue, including invasive carcinoma of the vagina, cervix, uterus, vulva, and penis.
3. HPV may be the most common STD in the United States, and estimates range between 5–20% of the sexually active population and close to 50% of sexually active college women.
4. HPV can be difficult to detect because there are often no clinical symptoms, and the virus can be localized internally on the genitalia.
5. There is no cure for genital warts, but they can be treated.
6. Pap smears should be done routinely to rule out cervical dysplasia and carcinoma.
7. Treatment includes cryotherapy, laser therapy, 5-fluorouracil and interferon.
8. Condoms are advised for patients with condyloma infection.

G. Syphilis
1. Syphilis is a venereal disease that has three recognized stages of development.
   a. The primary stage presents with a painless lesion or chancre that often goes unnoticed (particularly in women).
   b. If the infection is not cured at the primary stage, it progresses to secondary syphilis, which presents with a different set of highly infectious lesions.
   c. If untreated, the secondary stage will resolve and the disease will show no clinical signs for a long period of time (often many years) or may result in tertiary neurosyphilis.
2. Complications include irreversible destructive neurological signs and symptoms and congenital syphilis of neonates born to infected mothers.
3. The incubation of syphilis is about three weeks.
4. There has been a slow decline in the incidence of syphilis in the United States since 1947. The highest incidence is among poor, urban, heterosexual blacks.
5. Screening for syphilis is accomplished through serologic tests such as the Venereal Disease Research Laboratory (VDRL).
6. All patients with positive results should be interviewed for sexual history and encouraged to help locate those who may have been infected.
7. Treatment is typically a single IM injection of long-acting penicillin G.
8. Prevention and screening should be targeted to high-risk populations.

XV. **Prevention of Communicable Diseases**
A. Primary prevention
1. Primary prevention of communicable disease involves keeping the population healthy and free of contacting the disease.
2. Education of individuals, families, and aggregates at risk for a disease is an essential component.
3. Completion of schedule immunizations, elimination of high-risk sexual behaviors, clean needle programs, and programs that teach cognitive behavioral skills to address the social and cultural context of sexuality rather than behavior are examples of interventions.
B. Secondary prevention
1. Contact investigation, case finding, and screening are important secondary prevention

strategies to address and prevent the spread of communicable disease.
2. People whose sexual histories reveal high-risk behaviors should receive annual routine screening for STDs.
C. Tertiary prevention
  1. Keeping infected people away from those who are not infected
  2. Safely handling contaminated waste products
  3. Meticulous hand washing
  4. Wearing gloves when indicated
  5. Teaching family or other caregivers to give safe care to people in homes or institutions

TEACHING STRATEGIES

1. Obtain information from the state, county, and local health departments on reportable diseases in your area. Compare them with national rates provided in *MMWR*. Discuss why rates in your area are higher/lower than state and national rates. Where should interventions be focused?
2. Have students participate in immunization clinics.
3. Discuss universal precautions. How are they followed in clinical facilities and agencies where the students practice?
4. Monitor newspapers, magazines, and journals for communicable disease outbreaks locally, nationally, and worldwide. What has contributed to the outbreaks? What measures are being taken to limit their spread?
5. Invite a guest speaker from the STD or AIDS clinic at the local city or county health department. Encourage the speaker to discuss the most prevalent STDs in the community and identify at-risk groups. Have them discuss prevention strategies and how nurses can help define and diminish the problem.

CHAPTER 25

School Health

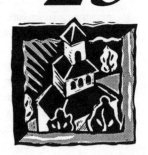

ANNOTATED LEARNING OBJECTIVES

1. Discuss the core components of school health in relation to roles and responsibilities of the multidisciplinary team.

Health care in the school is delivered to promote health and remove health barriers to learning. School health includes the interdependent components of school health services, school health education, and healthful school environment.

School health services include basic care (first aid and minor complaints), primary care, physical examination, screenings, and specialized care for children with disabilities or conditions specified in federal legislation. The responsibility for basic school health services largely rests on the nurse. Collaboration with physicians and other primary care providers and specialists (such as physical therapists, occupational therapists, and audiologists) is often necessary.

School health education is aimed at enhancing knowledge, attitudes, and behaviors that maintain and promote wellness and prevent or minimize disease. School health education may be provided by the nurse, a health teacher, public health personnel, or another specialist, such as an HIV educator.

A *healthful school environment* is considered critical to the health of students and is legally mandated in 40 states, although there is variation among states. School health environment includes the physical environment, psychosocial environment, and cultural environment. Team members who work to ensure a healthful environment include school administrators, nurses, teachers, and others.

Additional components of a comprehensive school health program are physical education, school food and nutrition services, guidance and counseling, school psychology, and work site health promotion. Interdisciplinary team members may include psychologists, counselors, dietitians, and physical education teachers.

2. Recognize the potential social, cultural, economic, and political factors affecting school health.

Factors that influence child health, and consequently school health, include problems such as poverty, low-birthweight infants, teen violence, out-of-wedlock teen births, juvenile incarceration, and poor high school graduation rates.

American children have the highest poverty rate of any group (more than 20% of American children grow up in poverty), and more than 9 million children had no health insurance in 1993. As a result, poor children have limited access to regular health care. Members of minority groups are particularly at risk and experience greater difficulty in seeking assistance for health care. The shift from two-parent to one-parent families and maternal employment affect many children, particularly minority children.

3. Relate community and statistical indicators of school health status to academic outcomes.

Poverty, poor health, and ethnicity influence school absenteeism, which in turn is associated with academic failure and dropping out of school. School-aged children miss an average of 3.8 days of school per year, but absenteeism is often much higher in children with chronic illnesses and in those without access to health care. Between 10% and 30% of all students have serious health problems, chronic illnesses, and/or impairments. Chronic illness may affect a child's ability to participate in regular school activities. A student who misses more than 11% of the school days during a semester has difficulty remaining at grade level.

4. *Apply the basic concepts of critical theory to school health.*

School health professionals should be actively engaged in identifying factors that prevent students from coming to school ready to learn, as well as factors that deprive them of access to resources that enhance their health and enrich the educational experience. To ensure that students have access to health-promoting choices, school health professionals should work to influence policy-making. By encouraging the support of funding for school health programs and the empowerment of individuals and groups to encourage autonomy and responsibility in addressing health care threats and health needs, school health professionals can prevent problems.

"Upstream thinking" with regard to school health programs can help ensure that students have access to health-promoting choices and come to school ready to learn. Efforts to define issues, raise consciousness, remove barriers, and facilitate change is essential to address current issues and problems.

5. *Formulate critical questions about school health programs that limit academic performance and well-being of school health populations.*

Social and health problems, along with fragmentation and inequity of health care services, challenge school health professionals to be creative in addressing sociopolitical issues in response to the needs of students. School nurses and others concerned with the health and well-being of school-aged children must be active in their efforts to improve student health and to address problems and potential problems that might adversely affect student health.

To formulate critical questions about school health, nurses should take the following steps.
1. Examine the context of an issue.
   • What is the history of the issue?
   • What efforts have been invested?
   • What will benefit a vulnerable groups?
2. Formulate a strategy to address the issue.
   • What resources are needed to resolve the issue?
   • What approaches would be effective?
   • How can the issue or problem be prevented in the future?
3. Implement the plan or strategy.
4. Evaluate the outcomes.

6. *Contrast roles and functions of school nurses and community health nurses.*

Like community health nurses, school nurses focus on health promotion and illness prevention interventions to individuals and aggregates. Their practice is ongoing, not episodic, and it takes place outside of the usual health care environment.

Unique characteristics of school nursing include a nursing practice based on generalist nursing knowledge regarding the entire life cycle and specialist knowledge of children and youth. School nursing is a solo practice; the nurse is usually the only health care professional in the school. The school nurse provides both episodic and long-term care within the time frame of the school year. School nursing practice requires professionalism, management principles, and interdisciplinary and interagency collaboration. The majority of school nurses are baccalaureate-prepared.

LECTURE OUTLINE

I. **A Critical Theory Approach to School Health**
   A. *School health* refers to programs that work to maintain and enrich the health of students, who comprise 20% of the U.S. population.
   B. School health professionals should be actively engaged in identifying factors that prevent students from coming to school ready to learn or deprive them of access to resources that enhance their health and enrich their educational experience.
   C. An "upstream approach" and a social justice philosophy are important to developing health promotion and illness prevention strategies to improve student health and solve problems that might interfere with learning.

II. **The Context of School Health**
   A. Modern school health began in the early 1800s in Great Britain and in the later half of the 19th century in the United States.
      1. The first school nurse was appointed in 1902 in New York City to achieve the following goals.
         a. Increase school attendance through health education
         b. Provide home visits for cases of communicable disease
         c. Improve hygiene
      2. Within 20 years, school health services had spread to more than 300 cities.
      3. Over the decades, additional services and foci have been added.
         1. Screenings
         2. Primary care and first aid
         3. Caring for children who have chronic illnesses and disabilities
   B. School health services have traditionally included three basic types of services.
      1. Delivering health services

2. Providing health education
3. Ensuring a safe school environment
C. Since 1985, increased enrollments and growth in numbers of children with disabilities or impairments have served to expand the need for comprehensive school health services.
D. Until recently, school health has been neglected as a potential avenue to influence children and youth.
   1. Policies that shape school health programs are established by state legislators.
   2. Many of the objectives from *Healthy People 2000* address issues related to children and school health.

III. **Indicators of School Health Status**
A. American children have the highest poverty rate of any age group.
   1. More than 20% of American children grow up in poverty.
   2. More than 9 million children had no health insurance in 1993.
   3. Poor children have limited access to regular health care.
B. Members of minority groups and the poor are particularly at risk, and they experience greater difficulty in seeking assistance for health care.
C. School absenteeism is associated with poverty, poor health, and ethnicity.
D. Between 10% and 30% of all students have serious health problems, chronic illnesses, or impairments.
   1. School-aged children miss an average of 3.8 days of school per year.
   2. Chronic illness may affect a child's ability to participate in regular school activities.

IV. **Components of School Health**—School health includes the interdependent components of school health services, school health education, and a healthful school environment.
A. School health services
   1. Health care in the school is delivered to promote health and remove health barriers to learning.
   2. School health services are mandated in 28 states.
   3. School health services include the following elements.
      a. Basic care (first aid and minor complaints)
      b. Primary care (acute and chronic complaints)
      c. Physical examination
      d. Screenings (vision, hearing, scoliosis, and other conditions)

   e. Specialized care for children who have disabilities or conditions specified in federal legislation (P.L. 94–142; P.L. 99–457; P.L. 101–476)
B. School health education
   1. Health instruction is aimed at enhancing knowledge, attitudes, and behaviors that maintain and enhance wellness and prevent or minimize disease.
   2. Most states have a comprehensive school health education program.
   3. School health education incorporates the following elements.
      a. Philosophy: Health education is based on beliefs about basing health education programs on local and global health priorities.
      b. Curriculum: Planned, sequentially developed content is delivered to students in kindergarten through grade 12 and is aimed at fostering individual responsibility and self care.
      c. Students: Recipients of school health education programs include school-aged children and youth, parents and family, teachers and others in the community.
      d. Evaluation: Ongoing assessment of programs requires input from school-aged pupils, teachers, school district personnel, and parents.
C. School health environment
   1. The general physical, psychosocial, and cultural environments are critical to health of students.
   2. A healthful school environment is legally mandated in 40 states, although there is variation among state requirements.
   3. School health environment includes the following elements.
      a. Physical environment: geographic location, school site and physical plant, air, temperature, lighting, noise, space, etc.
      b. Psychosocial environment: emotional and social conditions that influence students as well as staff interactions and activities
      c. Cultural environment: values, beliefs, ethnicity, language, policies that affect students, and staff communication and well-being
D. Additional components of a comprehensive school health program
   1. Physical education

a. Physical education enhances physical fitness and develops motor skills while promoting health through regular exercise and emphasis on a healthy lifestyle.

b. Physical education is legally mandated in 40 states.

2. School food and nutrition services

a. Food and nutrition services provide nutrition instruction and nutritionally adequate meals.

b. There is federal legislation regarding school lunches and breakfasts.

c. Thirty-two states have established a legal basis for a food service program.

3. Guidance and counseling

a. Guidance and counseling help students maximize their potential as members of society.

b. These services also ease the transition from grade to grade and help students explore career options.

c. Twenty-eight states have legislation for guidance and counseling.

4. School psychology

a. School psychology focuses on testing, placement, and clinical services.

b. Mainstreaming of children with impairments has expanded responsibilities to include special education screening and assessment.

5. Work site health promotion

a. Work site health promotion provides school faculty and staff with opportunities to address a growing awareness of the influence of health on learning.

b. Work site health promotion includes employee health examinations, health benefits, and wellness programs.

V. **School Health Financing**—School health programs consume less than 1% of public school expenditures. School health services are funded by the local school district, local health department, state education department, state health department, federal agencies, and voluntary philanthropy. Public schools are financed primarily through local and state sources.

A. State funding

1. Personnel is the largest expenditure in school health.

2. School health programs include an estimated 45,000 health professionals (30,000 nurses).

3. Costs vary greatly by state, depending on variations in state-mandated school health

programs, history, economics, demographic characteristics of pupils, and various interest groups.

4. Expenditures for public school health ranged from about $250 per student (Alaska) to $1.15 per student (Washington, D.C.).

B. Federal funding

1. Federal legislation provides some funding for health-related school programs for children with special needs

a. Services for the handicapped and disabled

b. Nutritional supplements

c. Protection from abuse

2. National child health policy is principally aimed at programs for handicapped and poor children and youth through the Maternal and Child Health Block Grant (Title V) and the Medicaid provision of the Social Security Act (Title XIX).

3. School environments are protected by several federal laws aimed at preventing and eliminating health hazards related to air and water quality, solid wastes, etc.

VI. **School Health Delivery Models**

A. Several models for school health programs are used throughout the United States.

B. The model used in a given school district depends on a number of factors.

C. Common models for school health programs include the following.

1. Mandated services are offered by the local public health department within health department budget limitations.

2. Public health services are combined with additional services purchased by the school district.

3. Health personnel are employed by the school district.

4. School-based health centers offer primary health care for students.

5. Full-service schools offer primary health care for students and their families.

VII. **The Practice of Nursing in the Schools**

A. Nurses are the primary health care providers in most schools.

B. School nursing includes many unique characteristics.

1. Practice is based on generalist nursing knowledge throughout the life cycle, with specialist knowledge of children and youth.

2. Emphasis is placed on health promotion, health maintenance, and disease prevention.

3. Practice is usually located outside of the usual health care environment (in schools, homes, or the community).
4. School nursing is often a solo practice; the nurse is usually the only health care professional in the school.
5. Care recipients are students, parents, groups, and aggregates.
6. Practice includes both episodic and long-term care within the time frame of the school year.
7. Practice requires professionalism, management principles, and interdisciplinary and interagency collaboration.
8. Most school nurses are baccalaureate-prepared.

VIII. Levels of Prevention

A. The school nurse's practice is based on preventing health problems that may interfere with students' education or with faculty and staff performance.
B. Interventions encompass all levels of prevention.
   1. Primary prevention
      a. Many interventions, such as immunizations, are mandated by law.
      b. Additional areas include educational programs to prevent substance abuse, STDs, or suicide.
      c. Health education teaches students about healthy lifestyles and the health care system.
   2. Secondary prevention
      a. Most states have mandated screening requirements for vision and hearing disorders and scoliosis.
      b. Height and weight monitoring, physical examinations before physical education and sports, and Early Periodic Screening, Diagnosis, and Treatment (EPSDT) are examples of other commonly performed screenings.

   c. Case finding is frequently utilized by school nurses to identify children with health care needs.
   3. Tertiary prevention
      a. Activities that correct or prevent further disability from a health problem are considered tertiary prevention.
      b. Caring for school children with chronic and handicapping conditions is mandatory in all schools.

IX. **Nursing Process**—School nurses must apply professional practice standards when working with students, families, and school personnel. The nursing process is the framework for this practice.

X. **Research in School Health**
   A. Researchers should examine the relationship between the school health system and related variables and outcomes.
   B. Researchers should document outcomes of various school health curricula.
   C. Teaching methodologies in health education should be examined.
   D. The implementation and impact of school health education on behaviors and student health should be examined.

TEACHING STRATEGIES

1. Invite a school nurse to speak to the class about school health programs and school nursing practice. Encourage the nurse to share a "day in the life of a school nurse" as illustrated in the chapter.
2. Have students share experiences they had with their school nurse during their elementary through high school years.
3. Assign a group of students to examine the impact of federal legislation, particularly P.O. 94–142, on school nursing. Have students debate the pros and cons of mandating that severely disabled children receive a public education. What is the subsequent impact on school nursing?

Environmental Health

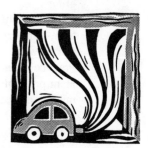

ANNOTATED LEARNING OBJECTIVES

1. Describe broad areas of environmental health about which community health nurses must be informed and name environmental hazards in each area.

Areas of environmental health and related health hazards of concern to community health nurses include:

- *Living patterns*—drunk driving, noise exposure, second-hand smoke, urban crowding, and stress
- *Work risks*—occupational poisoning, electrical hazards, motion injuries, presence of carcinogenic substances, and sexual harassment
- *Atmospheric quality*—destruction of the ozone layer, tornadoes, electrical storms, smog, herbicides, and acid rain
- *Water quality*—pollution by toxic chemicals, pathogenic microorganisms, oil spills, and lead leaching from pipes
- *Housing*—homelessness, fire hazards, dampness, rodent/insect infestation, lead-based paint chipping, and inadequate heating or cooling
- *Food quality*—malnutrition, bacterial food contamination, chemical additives, and improper meat inspection
- *Waste control*—poorly designed solid waste dumps, unlicensed waste dumps, inadequate sewage systems, and industrial dumping of toxic wastes
- *Radiation risks*—nuclear facility emissions, radioactive hazardous wastes, radon gas seepage, nuclear testing, and excessive exposure to medical and dental radiographs
- *Violence risks*—proliferation of handguns, hate crimes, violence in the media, and violent acts against women and children

2. Recognize potential social, cultural, economic, and political factors affecting environmental health.

The effects of the environment on public health are complex and often interconnected. Consequences of environmental hazards may be general or specific and may be immediate, long-range, or transgenerational.

Social factors that affect environmental health include transportation habits, pervasive violence, and waste control and management.

Cultural factors that influence health include diet and food preparation, living arrangements, family structure and roles, and religious practices.

Economic factors that influence environmental health include direct costs of cleaning up industrial waste and emissions; working in hazardous situations due to availability of employment; and costs related to research, testing, surveillance, monitoring, and evaluation of environmental risks.

Political factors that influence environmental health include special interest groups that often have power; governmental efforts to protect health, workers, and the environment; and conflicting social and economic groups that support opposing solutions to actual or potential problems.

3. Apply the basic concepts of critical theory to environmental health nursing problems.

Critical theory involves asking critical questions regarding the source of actual and potential threats to health that are observed in a community. The nurse must assess both immediate causes and environmental or social factors underlying these problems. The nurse must then choose sides and take a stand. Finally, the nurse must help mobilize vulnerable aggregates that are affected by the health threat and facilitate community involvement, form coalitions among affected community members and others interested in the problems, and use a variety of collective strategies to help change the environmental threat.

4. *Identify vulnerable aggregates that are at risk for particular environmental health problems.*

Vulnerable aggregates are those that are less able to protect themselves from pollution, inadequate housing, toxic poisoning, unsafe products, and other hazards. Racial minorities, children, the elderly, and illiterate manual laborers are some vulnerable aggregates in the United States.

5. *Distinguish between environmental health approaches that focus on altering individual behaviors and those that aim to change health-damaging environments.*

Approaches that place responsibility for the cause and cure of health problems exclusively on the individual absolves society, government, industry, and business for accountability for changing conditions under which people live and work. Many current efforts to improve health focus on altering individual behavior. Examples include efforts that encourage modifying lifestyles through exercise programs, smoking cessation, and stress reduction. This approach fails to include the broader environmental origins of disease, injury, and ecological destruction. Looking beyond the individual to recognize the environmental determinants of illness and wellness can be complicated and threatening. This approach involves social, economic, and political changes to improve the environment.

6. *Formulate critical questions about environmental conditions that limit the survival and well-being of communities.*

Critical questions assist in building collective strategies for problem resolution. When formulating critical questions, the nurse must assess how policies concerning ecological preservation, energy, housing, immigration, civil rights, crime, and so on are affecting the health and well-being of the people who live in the community. Critical questions about an actual or potential environmental threat might include:

- What is the problem?
- Who is defining the problem?
- What is the history of the problem?
- Who is affected by the problem?
- Who benefits from the way things are?
- Who has political power in the situation?
- What resources are needed to solve the problem?
- What are the barriers to health and relief from the problem?
- Who knows about the problem?

7. *Understand the skills needed to facilitate community participation and partnership in identifying and solving environmental health problems.*

The members of the community must participate in the process of identifying and working to solve environmental problems. Nurses must ask questions and help the community members determine how the environmental problems affect their lives. They should also be able to provide support, information, and expertise about the problem and its relation to health. Nurses can be instrumental in organizing coalitions of interested aggregates. They can organize forums, gather evidence, and meet with relevant businesspeople, health care providers, legislators, and members of the media.

8. *Propose collective strategies in which community health nurses can participate to address the environmental health concerns of specific aggregates.*

Strategies in which community health nurses can participate to address environmental health concerns include educational forums in neighborhoods; seminars for health care providers, city officials, teachers, and employers; community needs assessments; dissemination of clinical research using mass media; litigation; legislative lobbying and testimony at public hearings; demonstrations; and participatory research.

LECTURE OUTLINE

I. **A Critical Theory Approach to Environmental Health**

A. Helping communities become more aware of how the environment affects their health and helping them take actions to make needed changes in the environment is the ultimate goal of community health nursing.

B. Using critical theory, community health nurses should be vocally critical of conditions in the environment that affect the safety and well-being of aggregates or deprive them of access to resources necessary for the pursuit of health.

C. Use of critical theory can identify environmental sources of health problems.

1. Nurses should listen to what the community defines as problematic, help raise consciousness about environmental dangers, and assist in bringing about changes.

2. A critical perspective can help nurses plan and implement interventions at the aggregate level.

3. In assessment and analysis of environmental health, community health nurses should

always be aware of physical surroundings as well as the effects on communities of cultural realities, social relations, economic circumstances, and political conditions.

II. **Areas of Environmental Health**
  A. Living patterns
    1. Living patterns are the relationships among people, communities, and their surrounding environments that depend on habits, interpersonal ties, cultural values, and customs.
    2. Living patterns are not individual lifestyle choices, such as eating a high-fat diet or substance abuse, but they reflect population exposure to environmental conditions that are affected by mass culture, social practices, ethnic customs, and technology.
  B. Work risks
    1. Work risks include the quality of the employment environment and the potential for injury or illness posed by working conditions.
    2. Work risks pose the following environmental health problems.
      a. Sexual harassment
      b. Occupational toxic poisoning
      c. Electrical hazards
      d. Repetitive motion injuries
      e. Work sites containing carcinogenic particular inhalants such as asbestos and heavy metals
    3. Each year more than 20 million injuries and 400,000 illnesses are identified among American workers.
  C. Atmospheric quality
    1. Atmospheric quality refers to the protectiveness of the atmospheric layers, the risks of severe weather, and the purity of the air.
    2. Environmental dangers related to atmospheric quality include chlorofluorocarbon destruction of the ozone layer, forest destruction, tornadoes, electrical storms, smog, carbon monoxide, herbicides, and acid rain.
    3. Severe weather conditions can result in injury and loss of life, destruction of plants and wildlife, and property damage.
    4. Atmospheric pollutants can harm animals and plants and can cause lung cancer, chronic respiratory disease, and death.
  D. Water quality
    1. Water quality refers to the availability and volume of the water supply, mineral content levels, pollution by toxic chemicals, and presence of pathogenic microorganisms.
    2. Water quality consists of the balance between water contaminants and existing capabilities to purify water for human use.
    3. Problems of water quality include droughts, contamination of drinking supply by human wastes, pesticide-contaminated aquifers, lead leaching from water pipes, oil spills, water-borne bacteria, and excessive chlorination.
    4. Results of poor water quality may be an increase in water-borne diseases or problems brought about by toxic chemical pollution.
  E. Housing
    1. Housing refers to the availability, safety, structural strength, cleanliness, and location of shelter.
    2. The following environmental health problems are related to housing.
      a. Homelessness
      b. Fire hazards
      c. Inaccessibility for disabled people
      d. Illnesses caused by overcrowding, dampness, or rodent or insect infestation
      e. Chipping lead-based paint poisoning
      f. Injuries sustained from collapse of building structures
      g. Winter deaths from inadequate indoor heating
    3. Poor housing can spread infectious disease and can contribute to cardiovascular and respiratory disorders, cancer, allergies, and mental illnesses.
    4. The term *sick building syndrome* has been used to describe instances in which buildings and homes cause toxic symptoms in occupants due to building materials, poor ventilation, building operations, or substances in furniture, carpeting, or cleaning agents.
    5. The immediate environment in which the house is situated, including population density, proximity of industry, safety of adjacent buildings, level of security, and noise and pollution from nearby traffic, influences the housing environment.
  F. Food quality
    1. Food quality refers to the availability and relative costs of foods, their variety and safety, and the health of animal and plant food sources.
    2. Food quality problems include malnutrition, bacterial food poisoning, carcinogenic chemical additives, improper or fraudulent meat inspection, viral epidemics among

livestock, and food products from diseased animal sources.

3. Foods can be contaminated by toxic chemicals as they pass along the food chain and may result in reproductive and mutagenic effects in humans.

G. Waste control

1. Waste control is the management of waste materials that result from industrial and municipal processes and human consumption, as well as efforts to minimize waste production.

2. Several environmental health problems are related to waste control.
   a. Use of nonbiodegradable products
   b. Lack of efficient, affordable recycling programs
   c. Unlicensed waste dumps
   d. Inadequate sewage systems
   e. Industrial dumping of toxic wastes
   f. Coverups of illicit dumping
   g. Lack of enforcement of environmental protection legislation

3. The United States produces about 1 ton of waste per person per year.

4. Because of improper design, operation, or location of waste sites, hazardous substances may be spread through air, soil, and water to harm humans, plants, and animals.

H. Radiation risks

1. Radiation risks are the health dangers posed by the various forms of ionizing radiation.

2. Radiation risks include nuclear power emissions, radioactive hazardous wastes, medical and dental radiographs, radon gas in homes, and wartime use of nuclear weapons.

3. People living near nuclear facilities such as power plants, waste storage sites, and nuclear test sites have increased rates of cancers, strokes, diabetes, immune system damage, infertility, miscarriages, and birth defects.

4. Millions of Americans are exposed to dangerous levels of radon gas in their homes, schools, and workplaces. Radon seeps through basement walls, pipes, and foundation cracks and is trapped in buildings that have inadequate ventilation.

I. Violence risks

1. Violence-related environmental health problems can arise from conditions such as extreme poverty, widespread unemployment, proliferation of handguns, pervasive media images of violence, lack of child abuse services, and hate crimes.

2. Violent crimes include harassment, verbal abuse, battery, sexual assault, abduction, and murder.

3. Youth gangs, social stigmatization, political powerlessness of certain groups, and media images of male aggressiveness and sexual dominance reinforce cultural norms of violence.

4. Handguns, rifles, and automatic weapons are easily obtainable in the United States.

III. **Effects of Environmental Hazards**

A. Environmental effects on the public health are complex and often interconnected.

1. Nuclear power plant emissions can contaminate both water and air supplies.

2. Overcrowded housing may result in problems managing human wastes and may also perpetuate violent behavior.

B. Effects of environmental hazards may be general or specific, and they may be categorized as immediate, long-range, or transgenerational.

1. Examples of immediate effects include burns, gunshot wounds, hurricane damage, and food poisoning.

2. Examples of long-term effects include gradual occupational hearing loss, "black lung" disease in coal miners, and increased rates of cancer among migrant farm workers who are sprayed with pesticides.

3. Transgenerational effects may occur with radiation exposure of female factory workers at nuclear power plants or repetition of domestic violence in successive family generations.

IV. **Efforts to Control Environmental Health Problems**

A. The 1970s were the decade of environmental concern. New agencies designed to regulate environmental conditions at a national level were created by Congress.

1. Occupational Health and Safety Administration (OSHA)

2. Nuclear Regulation Commission (NRC)

3. Environmental Protection Agency (EPA)
   a. The EPA is responsible for protecting the environment and minimizing environmental risks to human health.
   b. The EPA sets standards for air and water quality; health surveillance and monitoring; evaluation of environmental risks; information acquisition; screening of new chemicals; and establishing, evaluating, and enforcing regulatory efforts.

B. In 1980, the EPA Superfund was established to clean up toxic sites.

C. There has been inadequate scientific research for formulating environmental health policy.

D. In general, most U.S. environmental health efforts have been directed by short-term goals rather than anticipating future needs and problems.

E. Nurses need to work with the public to set more stringent and actively enforced environmental regulations as well as greater social control over corporations and other groups that damage the environment.

V. **Approaching Environmental Health at the Aggregate Level**

A. In the United States, personal independence and individual responsibility for success and failure have always been very important.

1. Placing responsibility for the cause and cure of health problems exclusively on the individual reinforces the belief that all individuals are free to exert meaningful control over the quality and length of their lives.

2. This absolves society, government, industry, and business from accountability for changing conditions under which people live and work.

B. The current focus on interventions directed to the individual overlooks environments that "sicken" people.

1. Emphasizing only public health interventions to modify lifestyles through exercise programs, smoking cessation, and stress reduction fails to include the broader environmental origins of disease, injury, and ecological destruction.

2. Often changing individual behavior does not lead to significant reductions in overall morbidity and mortality in the absence of basic social, economic, and political changes.

3. Changes in basic social, economic, and political structure must be accomplished to improve the environment.

C. Looking beyond the individual to recognize the environmental determinants of illness and wellness can be complicated and threatening.

VI. **Critical Community Health Nursing Practice**

A. Taking a stand, choosing a side

1. Consequences of hazardous environments are often experienced inequitably.

a. Some vulnerable groups are exposed to more health-damaging effects than are less vulnerable groups.

b. Racial minorities, children, the elderly, and illiterate manual laborers are some of the groups in the United States who have little power to institute environmental change.

2. Decisions about the positions nurses accept and the interventions they undertake have the potential to increase or decrease these inequities.

3. Community health nurses have a mandate to assist vulnerable aggregates who are less able to protect themselves from pollution, inadequate housing, toxic poisoning, unsafe products, and other hazards.

B. Asking critical questions

1. Critical questioning can assist in building collective strategies for problem resolution.

2. The nurse must ask the following critical questions.

a. How do policies concerning ecological preservation, energy, housing, immigration, civil rights, crime, nutrition, minimum wage, occupational safety, and defense affect the well-being of people who live in the United States?

b. Who has access to resources in this country?

c. Whose interests are served by the current system?

C. Facilitating community involvement

1. It is essential that the members of the community participate in the process of identifying and working to solve environmental problems.

a. Nurses should join in mutual exchanges with community members.

b. Nurses must ask questions and help the community members determine how the environmental problems affect their lives.

2. The nurse should provide support, information, and expertise to assist the group in meeting their goals for environmental change.

3. The nurse can help the group members in looking beyond immediate environmental problems to explore social, cultural, economic, and political circumstances that affect them.

D. Forming coalitions

1. By building a strong basis of collective support, nurses can insist on structural changes that eliminate hazards and improve the public health.

2. Nurses can approach already existing community organizations and family and friendship networks to help mobilize aggregate members.

3. Nurses can be instrumental in organizing forums in which community groups can meet with scientific experts to gather evidence about health threats.

4. Nurses can meet with managers of businesses, heads of industry, and legislators to learn about problems and bring about change.

5. Press releases, media events, interviews, television spots, speeches, and newsletters can raise awareness among communities and call attention of outsiders to a situation.

E. Using collective strategies
   1. Nurses can use combinations of the following strategies to organize people to change health-damaging environments can be accomplished through combinations.
      a. Coalition building
      b. Consciousness-raising groups
      c. Educational forums in neighborhoods, workplaces, schools, churches, and social clubs
      d. Seminars for health care providers, city officials, teachers, and employers
      e. Community needs assessments
      f. Dissemination of clinical research
      g. Use of mass media
      h. Litigation
      i. Legislative lobbying and testimony at public hearings
      j. Demonstrations
   2. An effective aggregate-level community health nursing intervention is participatory research (action research).
      a. The goal of participatory research is the generation of open discussion and debate to intensify the community's awareness of how its health is affected by environmental constraints.
      b. Participatory research calls for nurses, community members, and other resource people to work together to iden-

tify environmental health problems that should be investigated.

c. They should help design the studies, collect and analyze data, disseminate results, and pose solutions to the problems.

d. The nurse helps the citizens gather data on suspected environmental hazards, document their effects on health, educate the community, persuade corporations to clean up, and lobby local, state, and federal governments for stricter regulations and better enforcement.

TEACHING STRATEGIES

1. Invite guest speakers such as
   - local city council or other community figures willing to discuss environmental health issues, policy matters, and ways to improve the environmental health of the community
   - local, county, or state public health nurses or occupational health nurses who work to decrease the impact of environmental health problems
   - officials from the EPA or NIOSH to discuss policy formation, standards legislation, compliance, regulation, and penalties with regard to environmental health issues

2. While in groups of three or four, have students choose one or two areas of environmental health described in the chapter (living patterns, atmospheric quality, food quality, etc.) and research a threat or potential threat in that area. Have each group answer the critical questions listed in Table 26-6 and discuss the results with the rest of the class.

3. Visit local groups or agencies that monitor, reduce, or seek to limit environmental health hazards. Examples include a local landfill, water treatment plant, public health department, nuclear power plant, or low-income or subsidized housing agency.

4. Identify actual or potential environmental health threats to individuals, families, or groups within the scheduled community health nursing clinical experience. Outline ways to reduce or eliminate these threats.

CHAPTER

27

Occupational Health Nurse: Roles and Responsibilities, Current and Future Trends

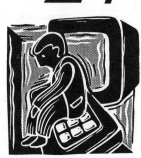

ANNOTATED LEARNING OBJECTIVES

1. *Describe the historical perspective of occupational health nursing.*

Occupational health nursing in the United States began in the late 1800s with the employment of Betty Moulder by a group of coal mining companies to care for miners and their families. Ada Mayo Stewart was hired about the same time to care for workers at a marble company and their families. During the early 1900s, the cost-effectiveness of providing health care to employees achieved recognition. The roots of occupational health nursing are entrenched in public health nursing practice, focusing on prevention, home care, and family-based health care.

In 1917, the first educational course for industrial nurses was offered at Boston University. The American Association of Industrial Nurses (AAIN) was begun in 1942. In 1953, the AAIN began publishing the *Industrial Nurses Journal,* and in 1977, the organization changed its name to the American Association of Occupational Health Nurses.

2. *Discuss the emerging demographic trends that will influence occupational health nursing practice.*

Several demographic changes will influence future occupational health nursing practice. U.S. industry is moving away from large manufacturing facilities to smaller service-based businesses. Flexible and varying work schedules and worksites will become standard. There will be a demand for an increase in the skill level of all employees and the ability to read, follow directions, and perform mathematic calculations will be required. An increase in the number of older workers, women, minorities,

and immigrants will affect employers and pose challenges for occupational health professionals. A shortage of workers is expected in the near future due to slow gains in the U.S. population growth rate.

3. *Identify the skills and competencies germane to occupational health nursing.*

Occupational health nurses should be able to direct care toward prevention of illness and injury and promotion of health. They must recognize and evaluate potential and existing health hazards in the workplace. Skills in areas of management and knowledge of toxicology, ergonomics, epidemiology, environmental health, safety, recordkeeping, budgeting, counseling, and education are essential to meet the present and future demand of occupational health nursing practice. Areas of responsibility include management and administration, direct care, health and environmental relationships, legal and ethical responsibilities, consultation, research, health education, and counseling.

4. *Apply the nursing process and public health principles to worker and workplace health issues.*

The occupational health nurse applies the nursing process through primary, secondary, and tertiary prevention strategies. Primary prevention includes both health promotion and disease prevention. Activities include development and implementation of aggregate-focused interventions such as weight reduction, AIDS awareness, ergonomics training, and smoking cessation. Health promotion strategies might include a health fair, on-site fitness center, stress management, and cancer awareness programs.

Secondary prevention includes identification of health needs, health problems, and clients at risk. Various types of health screenings, including tests for vision, cancer, cholesterol, hypertension, diabetes, and tuberculosis are used to identify early disease and encourage timely treatment.

Tertiary prevention strategies for the occupational health nurse include rehabilitation and restoration of the worker to an optimal level of functioning. Case management, negotiation of workplace accommodations, counseling, and support for workers who continue to be affected by chronic disease are some activities common in occupational nursing.

5. Discuss the role of state and federal regulations that impact occupational health.

Important federal regulations that impact occupational health include the Occupational Safety and Health Act and the Americans with Disabilities Act. The Occupational Safety and Health Act established the Occupational Safety and Health Administration (OSHA), which is responsible for promulgation and enforcement of occupational safety and health standards, and the National Institute of Occupational Safety and Health (NIOSH), which is responsible for funding and conducting research and making recommendations for occupational safety and health. The purpose of these organizations is to provide safe work sites and to protect the worker from death and serious harm.

The Americans with Disabilities Act prohibits discrimination on the basis of disability. This act requires employers to adjust facilities and practices for the purpose of making reasonable accommodations to enhance opportunities for individuals with disabilities. Workers' compensation acts are state mandated and state funded and provide income replacement and health care to workers who sustain a work-related injury, disability, or death. Workers' compensation acts protect the employer by precluding legal suits against the employer.

6. Describe a multidisciplinary approach to resolution of occupational health issues.

The occupational health nurse must recognize the need to work as part of an interdisciplinary team. The nurse must interact with occupational medicine professionals, industrial hygienists, safety professionals, employee assistance counselors, the personnel department, and union representatives. Community health professionals, insurance carriers, and other support agencies may also be involved in resolving occupational health issues.

LECTURE OUTLINE

I. **Definition of Occupational Health Nursing—**
The American Association of Occupational Health Nurses (AAOHN) defines occupational health

nursing as "the application of nursing principles in conserving the health of workers in all occupations. It emphasizes prevention, recognition, and treatment of illnesses and injuries and requires special skills and knowledge in the fields of health education and counseling, environmental health, rehabilitation, and human relations."

II. **Evolution of Occupational Health Nursing**
   A. The roots of occupational health nursing are entrenched in public health nursing practice, with a focus on prevention, home care, and family-based health care.
   B. The concept of occupational health nursing in the United States began in the late 1800s.
      1. Betty Moulder was employed by a group of coal mining companies to care for coal miners and their families.
      2. At about the same time, Ada Mayo Stewart was hired to care for workers at a marble company and their families.
   C. During the early 1900s, the cost-effectiveness of providing health care to employees achieved recognition.
   D. In 1917, the first education course for industrial nurses was offered at Boston University.
   E. The American Association of Industrial Nurses was begun in 1942.
      1. In 1953, the AAIN began publication of the *Industrial Nurses Journal.*
      2. In 1977, the organization changed its name to the American Association of Occupational Health Nurses.

II. **Roles of the Occupational Health Nurse**
   A. The role of the occupational health nurse is diverse and complex.
   B. The occupational health nurse works with workers, employers, and other professionals to identify health needs, prioritize interventions, develop and implement programs, and evaluate services.
      1. Ensure compliance with federal, state, and local regulations
      2. Develop health surveillance programs
      3. Counsel employees
      4. Coordinate health promotion and fitness activities
      5. Assess health and safety hazards in the workplace
      6. Establish comprehensive referral networks
      7. Manage occupational and non-occupational illnesses and injuries, including treatment of emergency and primary health problems
      8. Conduct health and safety evaluations

9. Perform case management of occupational and non-occupational illnesses and injuries
10. Consult with business and community partners
11. Manage various occupational health services, including program planning, policy development and analysis, budgeting, staffing, and general administration

C. Occupational health nurses are worker advocates, but they are also responsible to management.
   1. They must practice within a framework of company policies and guidelines.
   2. Ethical dilemmas may arise over issues such as drug screening, informing employees of hazardous exposure, and confidentiality.

D. Approximately 30,000 nurses (1.5–2% of all nurses) are practicing in occupational health settings in the United States. Over half of these nurses work alone, making decisions regarding health and safety issues, influencing policy on health and safety, and planning and implementing health programs.

E. Occupational health nursing includes several key practice areas.
   1. Health promotion and prevention
   2. Worker and workplace health hazard assessment and surveillance
   3. Primary care
   4. Research and illness or injury investigation
   5. Management and administration
   6. Community resourcefulness
   7. Legal and ethical issues

III. **Demographic Trends and Effects on Occupational Health Nursing**
A. Demographic trends that affect occupational health nursing
   1. U.S. industry is moving away from large manufacturing facilities to smaller, service-based businesses.
   2. Flexible and varying work schedules and work sites will become standard.
   3. There will be a demand for an increase in the skill level of all employees, and the ability to read, follow directions, and perform basic mathematic calculations will be required.
   4. An increase in the number of older workers, women, minorities, and immigrants will affect employers and pose challenges for occupational health professionals.
   5. A shortage of workers is expected in the near future due to slow gains in the U.S. population growth rate.

B. Increased emphasis on roles in prevention
   1. The median age of the U.S. workforce is getting higher as the workforce ages, and prevention must be increasingly emphasized to reduce the threat of chronic illnesses.
   2. The occupational health nurse uses strategies that are important in prevention and treatment of chronic disease.
      a. Primary prevention emphasizes health promotion and disease prevention. Interventions include smoking cessation, nutrition counseling, cardiovascular health education, fitness, and cancer prevention.
      b. Secondary prevention strategies in occupational health nursing include planning and implementation of health screening programs and performing health risk appraisals for early diagnosis and treatment of disease. Testing for cancer, hypertension, and cholesterol have been shown to be effective.
      c. Tertiary prevention strategies for occupational health nurses include the process of rehabilitation and encouraging employees to return to work following disability.
   3. Roles common to occupational health nurses include counselor, referral source, health educator, and consultant to management.

C. Women in the Workplace
   1. By 2000, approximately 47% of the workforce will be women, and 61% of U.S. women will be at work.
   2. Women's health and safety issues, including maternal-child health, reproductive health, breast cancer education and early detection, stress, and work-home balance issues will achieve increased significance.
      a. Working mothers—The occupational health nurse can play a key role in the development and delivery of prenatal, postpartum, and early childhood programs in the workplace. Employers must be educated regarding strategies to reduce health care costs for women and babies and to improve the work environment for mothers. Reproductive issues include exposure to chemicals know to be mutagenic or teratogenic.
      b. Breast cancer—Breast cancer is the second leading cause of cancer death among women (after lung cancer). Focus on

prevention begins with early detection. The occupational health nurse has an excellent opportunity to play a key role in reduction of morbidity and mortality associated with breast cancer by increasing breast cancer awareness and providing of accessible and affordable screening programs.

  c. Stress—Women may experience more stress than men in balancing their work and home roles. Child care issues continue to be primarily the responsibility of women, and women still handle most of the household responsibilities. Thus, women experience a unique form of stress. The occupational health nurse must be prepared to provide counseling and support for this problem. Educational programs and implementation of support groups will contribute to the health and productivity of these women.

D. Minorities in the workplace
  1. Over the next decade, minority groups will constitute an increasing share of the labor force.
  2. As the number of minority workers increases, so will illnesses traditionally associated with certain aggregates (heart disease and stroke, hypertension, cancer, cirrhosis, and diabetes).
  3. Minority workers are disproportionately represented in dangerous jobs and are at greater risk for developing occupation-related disease and injuries.
  4. The occupational health nurse, as an advocate, must negotiate with the employer for changes in the work environment to reduce or eliminate existing or potential harmful occupational exposures.

E. Delivery and access issues related to health care
  1. Increasing health care costs have produced a number of alternative approaches to providing health care.
  3. The occupational health nurse must be knowledgeable about the various health care options available to the workforce and the corporate benefits.
    a. Health maintenance organizations (HMOs) and preferred provider organizations (PPOs) are two of the more common health care management programs.
    b. Participation in one of the managed care plans requires that treatment take place

according to the organization's guidelines and within their health service delivery system.
    c. Access to care is strictly managed and often limited.
  6. As HMOs become more prevalent, the role of the occupational health nurse may take on added importance as a primary care provider.

F. AIDS in the workplace
  1. HIV infection poses a small but significant risk to health care workers.
  2. The occupational health nurse should educate and counsel workers with potential work-related AIDS exposure, as well as employees at risk because of personal behaviors.
  3. The occupational health nurse can influence employers to support workers with AIDS by improving benefits and making appropriate workplace modifications to allow work continuance.

G. AAOHN Year 2000 Recommendations—The AAOHN has submitted recommendations to help define the National Health Objectives for 2000.
  1. Provide convenient programs of monitoring, intervention, and follow-up for chronic illnesses by qualified occupational health professionals
  2. Educate at-risk workers about HIV transmission and self-protective measures
  3. Develop a company policy that protects at-risk workers while safeguarding the confidentiality and employment (as appropriate) of HIV-positive employees
  4. Offer voluntary, free, accessible vaccination against hepatitis B for health care workers at risk of blood exposure
  5. Provide health promotion and risk education programs by qualified occupational health professionals who are knowledgeable about occupational health issues as well as health promotion
  6. Encourage each state health department to hire at least one occupational health nurse consultant for local industries

IV. **Skills and Competencies of the Occupational Health Nurse**
A. Emergency care is an important part of occupational health nursing, but the current and future foci are on prevention of illness and injury and promotion of health.

B. The occupational health nurse must recognize and evaluate potential and existing health hazards in the workplace.
C. Skills in areas of management and knowledge of toxicity, ergonomics, epidemiology, environmental health, safety, recordkeeping, budgeting, counseling, and education are essential to meet the present and future demands of occupational health nursing practice.
1. Management and administration
   a. Managing budgets
   b. Hiring staff and managing staff performance
   c. Fostering professional development
   d. Developing program goals and objectives
   e. planning through knowledge of internal and external resources
   f. providing comprehensive on-site services and programs
   g. understanding needs of business and employees
   h. Writing reports
   i. Handling workers' compensation and disability
   j. Performing audits and quality assurance
   k. Performing cost-effectiveness and cost-benefit analyses
   l. Allocating staff resources
   m. Negotiating
   n. Facilitating work accommodations and return to work
   o. Coordinating medical response activities and site-disaster planning
2. Direct care
   a. Applying the nursing process
   b. Delivering first aid and primary care according to protocols
   c. Physical assessment
   d. History taking
   e. Medical testing
   f. Knowing immunization records
   g. Responding to medical emergencies
   h. Knowing trends in health-related issues
3. Health and environmental relationships
   a. Knowing plant operations, manufacturing processes, and job tasks
   b. Identifying potential and existing workplace exposures
   c. Influencing appropriate and targeted recommendations for control of hazards in the workplace
   d. Knowing toxicological, epidemiological, and ergonomic principles
   e. Understanding appropriate engineering controls, administration, and personal protective equipment specific to preventing exposure to health hazards
   f. Understanding roles and collaboration with other cross-functional groups as an integral part of a multidisciplinary team
4. Legal and ethical responsibilities
   a. Knowing AAOHN Professional Standards of Practice and Code of Ethics
   b. Knowing state nursing practice act and ability to practice occupational health nursing within state guidelines
   c. Knowing federal regulations pertaining to occupational health
   d. Knowing the Americans with Disabilities Act and related guidelines and Affirmative Action and Equal Employment Opportunity legislation
   e. Knowing medical recordkeeping practice in compliance with nursing practice, state law, and standards of practice
   f. Knowing current legal trends related to negligence and malpractice in professional nursing and in the occupational health setting
5. Consultation
   a. Being a resource expert on health issues for employees and management
   b. Having knowledge of public health and occupational health principles and practices
   c. Creating an effective professional and technical support network
6. Research
   a. Collecting, analyzing, and interpreting data from different sources
   b. Recognizing trends in health outcomes by department, work area, or workplaces
   c. Planning, developing, and conducting surveys
7. Health Education
   a. Recognizing cultural differences and the relationship to health issues
   b. Using effective communication styles to match diverse employee/management audiences
   c. Making effective presentations
   d. Planning, developing, implementing, and evaluating health programs designed to meet the needs of specific groups

e. Applying adult learning theories and principles to health education programs
8. Counseling
   a. Identifying employee's emotional needs and providing support and counseling
   b. Making appropriate referrals and/or recommendations
   c. Listening
   d. Managing psychiatric emergencies

V. Primary, Secondary, and Tertiary Levels of Prevention

—The occupational health nurse's practice is based on the concept of prevention. Goals set forth in the AAOHN's definition of occupational health nursing include promotion, protection, maintenance, and restoration of worker health.

A. Primary prevention
   1. In primary prevention, the occupational health nurse is involved in both health promotion and disease prevention.
   2. Primary prevention activities used by the occupational health nurse include developing and implementing aggregate-focused interventions such as weight reduction, AIDS awareness, ergonomics training, and smoking cessation.
   3. For health promotion, the nurse may plan and implement a health fair.
   4. The nurse may negotiate with the employer to set up an on-site fitness center or area with fitness equipment or to subsidize membership to a local fitness center.
   5. Other programs included in primary prevention include improving cardiovascular health, cancer awareness, personal safety, immunization, prenatal and postpartum health, accident prevention, retirement health, stress management, and relaxation techniques.

B. Secondary prevention
   1. The focus of secondary prevention is on identification of health needs, health problems, and clients at risk.
   2. By providing direct care for episodic illness and injury, the occupational health nurse has the opportunity to conduct early assessments and provide treatment and/or referrals for a variety of physical and psychological conditions.
   3. The occupational health nurse can offer health screenings at the work site.
      a. Vision
      b. Cancer
      c. Cholesterol
      d. Hypertension
      e. Diabetes
      f. Tuberculosis
      g. Pulmonary function
      h. Mammography
   4. Preplacement evaluation before the worker begins employment is often required.
      a. This evaluation offers a baseline examination consisting of medical history, occupational history, and a physical assessment.
      b. Medical tests to determine specific organ functions may also be required.
   5. Periodic assessments usually occur at regular intervals and are based on specific protocols for those exposed to substances or irritants such as lead, asbestos, noise, or various chemicals.

C. Tertiary prevention
   1. Occupational health nurses play a key role in the rehabilitation and restoration of the worker to an optimal level of functioning.
   2. Strategies include case management, negotiation of workplace accommodations, and counseling and support for workers who will continue to be affected by chronic disease.
   3. The occupational health nurse should be at the center of case management, and the nurse should work closely with the primary care provider to monitor the progress of the ill or injured worker and to identify and eliminate potential barriers to the process of returning to work.

VI. The Impact of Legislation on Occupational Health

A. The Occupational Safety and Health Act of 1970
   1. The passage of the Occupational Safety and Health Act came about because of worker health concerns, environmental awareness, union activities, increased knowledge about workplace hazards, and health concerns.
   2. The act requires employers to furnish a place of employment free from recognized hazards that may cause death or serious physical harm.
   3. The act identifies the roles of the various related government agencies, provides for the establishment of federal occupational safety and health standards, and identifies a structure of penalties, fines, and sentences for violations of regulations.
   4. The occupational health nurse must be knowledgeable about several components

of the Occupational Health and Safety Act. For example, the employer must keep records of work-related injuries, illnesses, and deaths.
5. The act formed several health-related organizations.
   a. *Occupational Safety and Health Administration (OSHA)* operates under the jurisdiction of the Department of Labor and is responsible for promulgating and enforcing occupational safety and health standards. OSHA has ten regional offices from which inspectors are assigned to enforce the standards and provide consultation to industries.
   b. *National Institute of Occupational Safety and Health (NIOSH)* operates under the jurisdiction of the Department of Health and Human Services and is responsible for funding and conducting research and making recommendations to OSHA for occupational safety and health standards.
   c. *Occupational Safety and Health Review Commission* is responsible for advising OSHA and NIOSH regarding legal implications of decisions or actions in the course of carrying out duties.
   d. *National Advisory Council on Occupational Safety and Health* is a consumer and professional organization that makes recommendations to OSHA and NIOSH regarding occupational health and safety.
   e. *National Commission on State Workers' Compensation Laws* existed to study the adequacy of state workers' compensation laws and to make recommendations. Their work ended in October 1972.
B. Workers' compensation acts
   1. Workers' compensation acts are mandated and funded by individual states, and each state regulates its own program.
   2. The purpose of workers' compensation acts is to provide income replacement and health care to workers who sustain a work-related injury.
   3. Workers' compensation acts also protect the employer by precluding legal suits against the employer.
   4. The employer can self-insure, contract with commercial insurance carriers, or purchase a policy with state-operated insurance funds.

5. Workers receive an average of 66% of their take-home pay before taxes, and some disabled workers and their families are also eligible for other benefits, such as Social Security.
6. The occupational health nurse can support both the employee and the employer in the area of workers' compensation.
   a. For the employee, the nurse may be the initial person to whom the work-related injury or illness is reported. Accurate assessment of the injury or illness and appropriate treatment are essential.
      1) The nurse may identify community resources so that the injured worker is provided with high-quality health care and appropriate medical follow-up.
      2) The nurse educates the employee regarding benefits under the workers' compensation act and is often the one who files the claim.
      3) If the employee is disabled for a period of time, the nurse provides case management, support, and remains in contact with the employee until return to work.
   b. For the employer, the nurse provides the expertise in early intervention and case management.
      1) The nurse's goal is to limit the worker's disability, while providing an opportunity for early return to work.
      2) The desired outcome is a productive employee with optimum health and productivity and reduced health care and workers' compensation costs.
C. The Americans with Disabilities Act (1991)
   1. The Americans with Disabilities Act prohibits discrimination on the basis of disability.
   2. The act requires employers to adjust facilities and practices for the purpose of making reasonable accommodations to enhance opportunities for individuals with disabilities.
   3. To meet the requirements of the act, the occupational health nurse must provide or facilitate reasonable accommodations and provide pre-employment health examinations.
   4. The examination must be job-related and consistently conducted for all applicants performing similar work.

VII. Professional Liability
   A. The occupational health nurse must know the legal parameters of practice and respond to legislative mandates that govern worker health and safety.
   B. Tensions may arise due to the nurse's responsibility to both the workers and the employer.

VIII. Multidisciplinary Teamwork
   A. The occupational health nurse must recognize the need to work as a part of an interdisciplinary team.
   B. The nurse interacts with occupational medicine professionals, industrial hygienists, safety professionals, employee assistance counselors, personnel, and union representatives. Community health professionals, insurance carriers, and other support agencies may also be involved.

TEACHING STRATEGIES

1. Invite an occupational health nurse from a local industry to speak to the class. Have the nurse include information about issues and roles commonly seen in occupational health nursing.
2. Invite a nurse from the employee health department of a local hospital to speak to the class. Ask the speaker to include information about safety issues in health care, including AIDS prevention strategies.
3. Divide the class into groups of two or three students. Have them complete the Preplacement Medical Evaluation, Occupational Health History, and Physical Demands Analysis provided in the text. If they are not currently working, have them hypothetically answer the question on physical demands based on clinical nursing experiences.

The Home Visit and Home Health Care

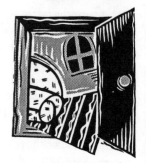

ANNOTATED LEARNING OBJECTIVES

1. *Discuss the purpose of the home visit.*

   The purpose of the home visit is to provide nursing care to individuals and their families in their homes. The focus of all home visits is the individual, but the nurse assesses the interaction of the individual with the family and provides education and interventions for the family as well as the client.

2. *Differentiate between the purpose of a public health nursing visit and that of a home health nursing visit.*

   The purpose of *public health nursing home visits* is to provide health education and primary prevention services. Public health nursing referrals are often for individuals and families who are poor and have no health care benefits. Antepartum or postpartum visits for high-risk individuals, followup of clients with communicable diseases, and care for clients in rural areas constitute most home visits for public health nurses.

   Home health nursing visits provide health care and social services for homebound or disabled individuals in their homes. Nursing services include assessment of physical, psychosocial, and functional needs. Care is short-term and intermittent and is based on the needs of the client. Often an interdisciplinary team approach is used, with the nurse serving as case manager. Home health nursing clients usually have health insurance which pays for the visits.

3. *Use the nursing process in outlining the steps involved in conducting a home visit.*

   Assessment
   - Prepare for the visit—review available information, obtain necessary equipment and supplies
   - Contact the client to set up an appointment
   - Assess the environment, including immediate community and neighborhood as well as the home
   - Begin the visit with social conversation to establish a comfortable atmosphere and build trust
   - Perform a physical assessment—review all systems, emphasizing the affected system
   - Perform a functional status assessment—observe the client's ability to perform activities of daily living

   Diagnosis and Planning
   - Develop a plan of care for the client and family
   - Verify the plan of care with the client
   - Identify goals (should be accomplished with the client/family)
   - Outline roles of the nurse, client, and family

   Intervention
   - Provide information concerning the client's health status
   - Profind information concerning community resources
   - Provide skilled nursing care when needed
   - Provide referrals for other services
   - Discuss the need for further visits and schedule visits accordingly
   - Terminate the visit

   Evaluation
   - Evaluation is continuous throughout client contact
   - Input from client is obtained on progress toward identified goals
   - Plans are modified as needed
   - When goals are achieved and nursing interventions are no longer needed, the relationship is terminated

4. Define home care.

Home health care describes a system in which health care and social services are provided to homebound or disabled people in their homes rather than in medical facilities. Services in home health include care provided by registered nurses, physical therapists, occupational therapists, speech therapists, social workers, and home health aides.

5. Identify the types of home health agencies.

Types of home health agencies include official agencies (agencies operated and funded by local or state governments); nonprofit agencies (agencies exempt from paying federal taxes); proprietary or "for profit" agencies; home health chains (agencies owned and operated by corporations, usually proprietary); and hospital-based agencies.

6. Discuss the process used in contracting with patients and their families to achieve health care goals.

Following identification of health needs and verification of those needs with the client, a plan of care for the client and the client's family is developed. The nurse assists the client in identifying goals toward which the client is willing to work. A contract is developed to delineate the role and responsibilities of the nurse and the role of the client and family. The written contract can be used as a reference and may be modified by mutual agreement.

LECTURE OUTLINE

I. **Home Health Care**—*Home health care* describes a system in which health care and social services are provided to homebound or disabled people in their homes rather than in medical facilities.

II. **Purpose of Home Health Services**
   A. Home health services allow individuals to remain at home and receive health care that would otherwise be offered in a health care institution (hospital or nursing home).
   B. The home health industry has grown tremendously over the past decade due to increasing costs of hospital care and introduction of the prospective payment system, and subsequent use of DRGs.
      1. This change in the reimbursement system has provided motivation for hospitals to improve their utilization to better control patient length-of-stay.
      2. As a result, patients are discharged from hospitals with the need for continuing intermittent health care, and are therefore candidates for home health services.

III. **Conducting a Home Visit Using the Nursing Process**
   A. Visit preparation
      1. The nurse prepares by reviewing the referral form and other available information.
      2. Information from the referral form should include name, age, diagnosis or health status, purpose of the visit, address, telephone number, insurance if any, medication, diet, reason for referral, and source of the referral.
   B. The referral
      1. A referral is a formal request for a home visit.
      2. Referrals come from hospitals, clinics, health care providers, individuals, and families.
         a. *Home health* referrals are requested to provide short-term, intermittent skilled services and rehabilitation to clients. Dressing changes, IV therapy, and diabetic education are examples.
         b. *Public health* referrals are made for clients who need health education (infant care, family planning) or for followup of clients with communicable diseases or their contacts.
   C. Initial telephone contact
      1. The client is contacted by the nurse and is informed of the referral for service.
      2. The nurse should introduce him- or herself, identify the agency, discuss the purpose of the visit, receive permission, and set a time and place for the visit.
      3. If the client does not have a phone, the nurse may choose to make a drop-in visit.
   D. Environment
      1. An environmental assessment should be done, reviewing the neighborhood, shopping facilities, transportation, etc.
      2. The client's dwelling is assessed.
         a. Accessibility by the client
         b. Handicapped facilities, if necessary
         c. Security
         d. Whether the client lives alone
         e. Source of nutrition
         f. Presence of vermin
         g. Running water
         h. Heat/cooling
         i. Sanitation facilities
         j. Whether the home is cluttered with debris and furniture
   E. Safety issues
      1. If the nurse does not feel safe entering a client's home environment, the nurse should not enter but call the client and make other arrangements.

2. No nurse is expected to disregard personal safety in an effort to make a home visit.

F. Building trust
   1. It is not uncommon for a client to mistrust the health care system.
   2. A trusting relationship should be built early in the visit.

IV. Application of the Nursing Process

A. Assessment
   1. The type of assessment varies depending on the purpose of the home visit.
      a. *The public health nurse* assesses the client's knowledge of his/her health status and identifies knowledge deficits. Subjective information, client perceptions of the problem, family network, and social support will be assessed.
      b. *The home health nurse* assesses the client's health knowledge and performs a physical assessment. The assessment includes a review of all systems, with an emphasis on the system affected by the client's presenting condition.
   2. Observation, palpation, auscultation and percussion should be used to collect objective data.
   3. Assessment of the functional status of the client is very important.
      a. This includes information regarding the client's ability to ambulate, to perform activities of daily living independently, and to use assistive devices such as a cane or wheelchair.
      b. Functional limitations such as shortness of breath or muscle weakness are also assessed.

B. Diagnosis and planning
   1. Develop a plan of care for the client and family
      a. A plan of care for the client and family is based on identified needs.
      b. These needs should be verified with the client and family.
      c. Mutual goals are identified.
      d. An important goal for home visits is to encourage the client to take an active role in health promotion. The nurse must work to ensure that the client does not become dependent on the nurse's interventions.
   2. Outline the client and family roles
      a. The nurse might use written contracts outlining the client's and nurse's roles in implementation of the plan.

      b. The contract may be modified at any time by mutual agreement of the client and the nurse.

C. Intervention
   1. Implementation of the care plan begins during the first home visit.
   2. The nurse provides the client and family with health information concerning the client's health status and availability of, and access to, community resources.
   3. In a home health visit, the nurse provides skilled nursing care.
   4. At the end of the visit, the nurse discusses the need for additional visits.

D. Referral for community services
   1. During the first visit, the nurse provides the client and family with information about community resources, including services provided, eligibility, and telephone numbers.
   2. Referrals depend on the availability of community resources, eligibility of the client, willingness of the client to use the resources, and suitability of the resources for the client.
   3. The client and family are encouraged to make the contacts, but if they are unable or unwilling, the nurse may intervene.

E. Terminating the visit
   1. The nurse terminates the visit when the assessment is completed and a plan for care is established.
   2. The average first visit should not last more than an hour.
   3. A date for the next visit, if required, is set.

F. Evaluation
   1. Evaluation of progress toward goals is continuous, and allows the nurse to determine the success of or progress toward goals.
   2. Input from the client is critical to determine whether the goals are realistic and achievable.
   3. Evaluation allows the nurse and client or family to discuss what is working well and where modifications in the plan are needed. Good communication is essential.
   4. The purpose of home visits is to assist the client with the information and nursing care that is necessary to function successfully without interventions by the nurse. When the goals have been achieved, the nurse is no longer needed by the client.

V. Types of Home Health Agencies

A. Official agencies
   1. Official, or public, home health agencies are organized, operated, and funded by local or state governments.

2. These agencies may be part of a county health nursing service or a home health agency that operates separately from the public health nursing service.
3. Official home health agencies are funded by taxpayers as well as third-party payers such as Medicare, Medicaid, and private insurance companies.

B. Nonprofit agencies
1. Nonprofit home health agencies are those agencies that are exempt from paying federal taxes because of their tax status and because they reinvest their profits into the agency.
2. Nonprofit home health agencies include independent home health agencies and hospital-based home health agencies (although not all hospital-based agencies are nonprofit organizations).

C. Proprietary agencies
1. Proprietary home health agencies are those classified as 'for profit"; these agencies pay federal income tax.
2. Proprietary agencies may be individually-owned agencies, partnerships, or corporations.

D. Chains
1. A growing number of home health agencies are owned and operated by corporate chains.
2. These chains are usually classified as proprietary agencies and/or may be a part of a proprietary hospital chain.

E. Hospital-based agencies
1. The number of hospital-based agencies has grown dramatically during the last decade due to fixed reimbursement.
2. Establishment of home health agencies allows hospitals to discharge patients who still have health care needs, provide necessary services, and receive reimbursement.
3. The increasing number of home health agencies indicates that home health care is profitable and provides hospitals with a source of additional revenue.

F. Certified and noncertified agencies
1. Certified home health agencies meet federal standards and are therefore able to receive Medicare payments for services provided to eligible individuals.
2. Only about half of all agencies are certified.

G. Special home health programs
1. Many home health agencies offer special, high-technology home care services.

2. Offering high-technological services at home is beneficial for the patient and iis financially advantageous.
3. Patients who require continuous skilled care in acute or skilled nursing institutions are able to return to their homes and receive care.
4. Examples of special services
a. Home intravenous therapy for patients who require daily infusions of total parenteral nutrition or antibiotics
b. Pediatric services for children with chronic heath problems
c. Followup of premature infants
d. Ventilator therapy
e. Home dialysis
5. The key to success of special home health care is the patient's, family's, or caregiver's ability and motivation to learn the care. If family or caregiver support is not available in the home, the patient is not a candidate for these programs and other arrangements for care must be made.

H. Reimbursement for home care
1. Since 1965, individuals who are eligible for Medicare or Medicaid, and those with private health insurance, can receive short-term skilled health services in their homes that are reimbursed by the federal government.
2. Services provided include nursing care, social services, physical therapy, occupational therapy, and speech therapy.
3. Public sources finance about 75% of home health care, more than half of which is paid by Medicare. The remainder is paid by a combination of out-of-pocket payment and insurance.
4. The rapid growth of the home health market is believed to be due to the increasing proportion of people age 65 or older, lower average cost of home care compared with institutional care, active support of insurers for home care, and Medicare promotion of home health care as an alternative to hospital care.

VI. **Educational Preparation of Home Health Nurses and Nursing Standards**
A. The ANA has established standards for home health nursing practice divided into two levels.
1. Generalist home health nurse
a. The generalist home health nurse is prepared at the baccalaureate level.
b. The generalist provides care to individuals and their families and must have

community health assessment skills to diagnose complex biopsychosocial problems in families, teach health practices, counsel, and refer to other health care providers as necessary, as well as perform high-tech nursing skills.
  2. Specialist nurse
    a. The specialist nurse is prepared at the graduate level.
    b. The specialist home health nurse has additional clinical expertise and may formulate health and social policy and implement and evaluate health programs and services.
B. Program requirements for home health nurses
  1. Nursing programs at the undergraduate and graduate levels that prepare competent providers of home health care
  2. Curricula that include concepts related to the health service system and the home subsystem
    a. Structural, process, and outcome elements
    b. A minimum of one clinical observation or experience in a home health care agency for undergraduate students
    c. specific courses at the graduate level that cover concepts such as education, prevention, therapeutic and high-tech nursing interventions for home health care, multidisciplinary approach to home health care, health law and ethics, systems theory, economies, and case management.

VII. Documentation of Home Care
A. Documentation typically provides the source of greatest frustration for home health nurses.
  1. Because of the influence of Medicare, regulations stipulated by the Health Care Financing Administration determine the home health industry's documentation.
  2. Correct and accurate completion of all required forms is necessary for reimbursement.
  3. Payment or denial for visits made is based on the information that is presented on the required forms. If the nurse does not clearly document in the nursing notes the skilled care that is provided, the fiscal intermediaries will argue that the care was either not necessary or not done, and reimbursement will be denied.
B. Documentation of care to record the quality of care received by the patient is also very important.

1. Documentation of the home visit serves as the record of the nurse's observations and assessment of the patient's condition
2. It also provides a record of interventions and of the ability of the patient and family to manage the care at home.
3. Documentation also serves as formal communication among other home health professionals who have interactions with the patient and family.

VIII. The Family or Caregiver in Home Care
A. The family member or caregiver makes the difference between the successful or unsuccessful completion of the plan of treatment.
B. The home health nurse often spends much of the visit assessing the skills of the caregiver.
C. The caregiver is instructed by the home health nurse in the correct procedures for providing care and in recognizing the signs and symptoms of problems.
D. The goal of the nurse's instruction is to provide the caregiver with the skills necessary to care for the patient in the home without intervention by the nurse or other members of the home health team.
E. When the patient lives alone and does not have caregivers, the nurse explores other resources available to supplement the patient's self-care activities in the home.

IX. Hospice Home Care
A. Characteristics of hospice home care
  1. Home care for the terminally ill has two goals.
    a. To keep the client comfortable at home as long as possible
    b. To provide support and instruction to caregivers.
  2. When the patient has been determined to be dying, the focus changes from cure to comfort.
  3. It is vital to realize that caring for the terminally ill includes caring for the family.
  4. When caring for a terminally ill person at home, the hospice nurse must be skilled in physical and psychosocial care for both the patient and the caregiver.
  5. The patient is viewed as a whole person, not as an isolated disease.
B. Caring for the caregiver
  1. Although the dying patient is the focus of hospice nursing care, careful assessment of the caregivers' mental and physical health is important.

2. The spouse, children, friends, and neighbors who have made the commitment to stay until the end need the nurse's time and attention as much as, if not more than, the patient.
3. Although the wishes of the patient are important, all decisions regarding care are made with the health of the caregivers in mind.
C. Pain control and symptom management
  1. The avoidance of peaks and valleys in pain management by building a wall against pain was begun in the United States about 15 years ago.
  2. In hospice nursing, pain medication is given on a regular schedule to prevent pain from recurring and is given in doses sufficient to keep the patient pain-free. The vast majority of patients can be pain-free until their deaths.

3. The key to successful pain control for the terminally ill is to convince patients to take their medications on a regular basis, not just when they can't stand it any longer.

TEACHING STRATEGIES

1. Invite a home health nurse and a public health nurse to be guest speakers. Have each explain how referrals for their services are obtained. Encourage an outline of the process of a typical home health visit. What type of clients does each generally see? What is the source of payment for services? How are visits and care documented?
2. Arrange for one or two students to accompany a public health nurse on a home visit, and for one or two to accompany a home health nurse. Have each group report back to the class on their observations.

World Health

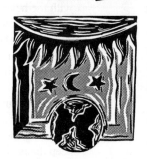

ANNOTATED LEARNING OBJECTIVES

1. *Identify three forces that threaten life and health worldwide.*

   Exponential population growth increases malnutrition and violence. It also threatens health and the economy in developing nations. Dense living arrangements promote stress and the transmission of communicable disease.

   Environmental stressors directly assault human health, damage society's goods and services, damage the quality of life, and interfere with ecological balance and other forms of life, thus influencing health worldwide.

   Disease patterns in both developed and developing countries affect health and threaten life. In developed countries primary causes of death include cardiovascular disease, cancer, respiratory disease, stroke and violence. In developing countries primary causes of mortality are infectious diseases (hepatitis B. rheumatic heart disease, malaria, measles, polio and tuberculosis), malnutrition and violence.

2. *Compare and contrast Cuba's and Canada's approaches to the delivery of primary health care.*

   In Cuba, health care services are provided by the government and are available to all citizens without cost. Health care services are community-based, population-focused, comprehensive, and delivered within a geographic base. The basic model for delivery of primary health care is the family medicine or neighborhood/home clinic. Health promotion and primary prevention are stressed. The family physician and nurse live in the community in which they practice in a combination home/clinic. Health education focuses on health promotion programs for groups in the community.

   Similarly, in Canada, health care services are provided by the government (at the provincial level) and are available to all citizens at no cost. However, the structure is a government-financed health insurance model. The provincial insurance plans are individual-focused and include universal coverage, portability of coverage from province to province, comprehensive coverage for all in-hospital care, reimbursement for physician's services, accessible services, and a publicly administered plan. In general, although the Canadian system has removed direct financial barriers to accessing hospital and physician service, it has retained a fee-for-service payment method for medical care that is biased against preventive activities.

3. *Describe Cuba's model of population-focused nursing.*

   Population-focused nursing is characterized by science-based nursing care delivery; interventions directed at the population or subpopulation level; focus on more than one subpopulation; attention to those in need who do not seek care as well as those who do; and concentration on matching the health needs of a community and its resources.

   In Cuba, community health nursing practice integrates a population focus, mobilization of the community for health, primary care, community health care, and home health care. It is comprehensive and is practiced within a geographic base.

LECTURE OUTLINE

Community health nurses must be aware of forces that threaten health around the world. They should study models of health care delivery in other countries that may promote the well-being of the greatest number of people. Health issues that demand attention and study include population growth, environmental stressors, and disease.

A. Population Growth
  1. Large populations create pressure.
     a. In developing countries, feeding a population may be a problem.
     b. Malnutrition, disease, or death may be the outcome.
  2. World population growth is often overlooked as a health-related problem, yet current, rapid growth presents a threat to the health and economy of many nations.
  3. Population growth has increased exponentially from 1 billion around 1800 to 2 billion in 1927, 3 billion in 1960, 4 billion in 1974, and 5 billion in 1987. It is estimated to reach 6 billion by 1998 and 7 billion by 2005.
  4. Distribution of population is uneven, with 52% of the people living in five countries: China, India, the former Soviet Union, the United States, and Indonesia.
  5. As the world's population grows, there is a rising trend toward urbanization, with people living closer together. Increasingly, dense living arrangements threaten the health of the general population and cause environmental stress.

II. **Environmental Stressors**
  A. Types of environmental stressors
    1. Stressors that directly assault human health, such as lead poisoning
    2. Stressors that damage society's goods and services, such as air pollution
    3. Stressors that damage the quality of life, such as litter and noise
    4. Stressors that interfere with ecological balance and other forms of life, such as water pollution, solid waste, and radiation.
  B. Patterns of Disease
    1. Disease patterns and the primary causes of mortality differ in developed and developing countries.
       a. In developed countries, primary causes of mortality include cardiovascular disease, cancer, respiratory disease, stroke, and violence (motor vehicle accidents, homicide, suicide).
       b. In developing countries, primary causes of mortality are infections, malnutrition, and violence.
       c. Infectious diseases frequently found in developing countries include hepatitis B, rheumatic heart disease, malaria, measles, polio, and tuberculosis.

  2. AIDS is shared globally, although there is considerable geographic variation in factors such as gender differences and modes of transmission.
  C. Promoting health in developing countries
    1. Promoting health worldwide is a great challenge.
    2. The World Health Organization (WHO) created a program of low-technology health care to prevent disease in poor countries. The program is prevention-based and designed to take most health care out of urban areas and disperse it throughout the communities.
    3. The goal of health for all may be achieved through cleaner air, improved nutrition, clean water, sanitation, vaccination, contraception, essential drugs, and mother and child health care.
  D. Promoting health in developed countries
    1. Health care systems in developed countries, which are heavily dependent on specialized medical technologies, are not appropriate models for developing countries.
    2. The health care policy in many developed countries fails to make health care available to the general public.
    3. Medical costs increase annually, and citizens are faced with paying increased amounts for health care.
    4. Because of the market-based economy, health care is seen as a commodity to be bought and sold, and focuses on curative medicine rather than prevention.
    5. Nursing should seek to implement and establish a population- or community-based, rather than market-based, health care system to meet the needs of the population.

IV. **Primary Care in Cuba**
  A. The World Health Organization's definition of primary health care—According to WHO, primary health care should include the following.
    1. Universal coverage
    2. Relevant, acceptable, affordable, and effective services
    3. Comprehensive services providing primary, secondary, and tertiary care and prevention
    4. Community involvement in planning and delivery of services
    5. Integration of health services with development activities to ensure that complete nutritional, educational, occupational, environmental, and safe housing needs are met.

B. History of the development of Cuba's primary health care model
  1. Cuba is a small, developing country. After the revolution in 1959, primary health care, which was largely not available to the masses, became available to all through community organizations.
  2. This resulted in improved sanitation, immunizations and construction of roads, housing, hospitals, clinics, and medical and nursing schools.
C. Cuba's neighborhood/home clinics
  1. Beginning in 1984, family medicine or neighborhood/home clinics became the standard model for delivery of primary care.
  2. Understanding, integration, coordination, and administration of care of the individuals, families, and community became the foundation of medical education.
  3. The family physician and nurse live in the community in which they practice in a combination home/clinic.
  4. Clinic hours are held in the mornings, and both the nurse and the physician make home visits during the afternoon.
  5. Health education focuses on health promotion programs for groups in the community.
D. Achievements in health as a result of Cuba's model
  1. Due to improvements in health care delivery, morbidity and mortality rates are similar to, and sometimes better than, those in developed countries.
  2. Cuba has been recognized as achieving "Health for All" with equity in health services that has no class or racial differences.
E. Consequences of Cuba's model for women's health
  1. Cuba has remarkably decreased its infant mortality rate since the revolution.
  2. More than 95% of pregnant women begin receiving prenatal care in the first three months of pregnancy, and all women are seen at least monthly during pregnancy.
  3. Every child under one year of age is seen monthly, and home visits are made to assess the infant's development.
  4. Sex education and contraception are available.
  5. One concern, however, is that due to the availability of abortion, many women use abortion as birth control, and rates are very high.
F. Effects of the "special period" of economic hardship on Cuba's health care model

  1. Since 1991, serious economic difficulties have impacted Cuba.
  2. As a result, essential food items such as meat and milk have been rationed, and economic hardships have taken their toll.
  3. Alternative medicines have been used to alleviate the shortage of medicines.
  4. There has been a concurrent lack of exchange of professional literature in the health field.
  5. Lack of trade has affected the availability of medical and nursing journals and, as a result, other countries have little knowledge of Cuba's innovative health care system.
G. A critique of Cuba's model
  1. Criticisms of Cuba's health model include concern over the following problems.
    a. Massive expenditures on health when there is concurrent rationing of basic food items
    b. Little petroleum for fuel and industrial use
    c. Large expenditures for some medical programs (such as comprehensive residential care for HIV+ patients) at the expense of other programs (such as ensuring a safe water supply)
  2. Smoking is still a major problem, seatbelts are not used, and exercise is not largely valued.
  3. The Cuban diet is high in fat and low in vegetables.

V. **Primary Health Care in Canada**
  A. Characteristics of Canadian health care
    1. Geographically, Canada is very large; however, the population is relatively small and tends to be concentrated near the U.S./Canadian border.
    2. Since 1950, life expectancy has increased almost eight years for men and ten years for women.
    3. Infectious diseases have declined significantly.
    4. The leading causes of mortality are typical of industrialized nations (cardiovascular disease, cancer, respiratory disease, strokes, and accidents).
  B. Emergence of a universal health care system
    1. In 1867, the Canadian government assigned the responsibility of health of the citizens to the provincial governments.
    2. Commercially-based insurance plans similar to those that developed in the United States began in the 1930s.

3. Considerable variation existed among the provincial plans, and many people found themselves ineligible for the plans or unable to meet premiums.
4. The first universal hospital insurance plan was instituted in 1947 in Saskatchewan. Every resident was required to register for the plan, which was subsidized by general tax revenues. Other provinces soon followed.
5. These plans included the following features.
   a. Universal coverage
   b. Portability of coverage from province to province
   c. Comprehensive coverage for all in-hospital care
   d. Accessible services
   e. Publicly administered plan
   f. In 1968, reimbursement for physicians' services was added to provincial health insurance plans.
7. In general, although the Canadian system has removed direct financial barriers to accessing hospital and physician service, it has retained a fee-for-service payment method for medical care that is biased against preventive activities.
C. Changing paradigms for health care delivery
   1. In 1974, it was noted that lifestyle and environment issues shifted health care away from the traditional medical model to a more holistic system-environment perspective.
   2. The Ottawa Charter for Health Promotion, Health, and Welfare (1986) provided a health promotion framework with the following goals.
      a. Fosters public participation in processes and decisions that affect health
      b. Strengthens community health services by improving links between services and the communities they serve
      c. Coordinates public health policy so that professionals in public policy arenas become aware of their interest in, and responsibility toward, health in their communities
D. Rising cost of health care
   1. In the 1980s and 1990s, the rising cost of health care has served to change health care delivery.
   2. In 1992, health care cost in Canada accounted for 11% of the GNP (up from 7% in 1970).
   3. Reform efforts are underway in many provinces to increase efficiency of service.

E. Transitions in community health nursing
   1. Community and public health nurses in Canada have had an important role in health care delivery in Canada since the early 1900s. Services provided by public health nurse include the following.
      a. Home visiting
      b. Group work
      c. Well-baby care
      d. Prenatal classes
      e. Health promotion programs
      f. Other health programs
   2. Attempts to find more cost-effective ways to deliver public health services in response to demographic changes (aging population, minority needs) has resulted in changes in emphasis such as such as the following.
      a. A shift in focus from family care programs to initiatives with groups
      b. Increasing the range and diversity of community interventions (i.e., coalition formation, community development, and health policy development)
      c. Increasing emphasis on population-based approaches and working with the hard-to-reach clients rather and managing the followup of clients referred by the health care system.
F. Articulating new roles for the community health nurse in Canada
   1. Many Canadian nursing associations have recognized the need to promote primary health care within their provincial governments.
   2. They have recommended several changes to meet this need.
      a. Place a priority on health promotion and illness prevention by addressing underlying causes of illness and integration of primary health care principles at the primary, secondary, and tertiary levels
      b. Recognize the importance of a multidisciplinary approach that links referral mechanisms, incorporation of a multifaceted approach to health promotion, including education, training, research, lobbying, community mobilization, and development of community partnerships
      c. Provision of services that are financially, geographically, socially, and culturally accessible with multiple points of entry.
G. Innovative Health Care Delivery Models
   1. Teaching Health Units

a. Initiated in the 1980s, the Teaching Health Units were established by the Province of Ontario to address health needs through education, research, and clinical practice.
b. Examples of their work include research on the impact of follow-up home visits for postpartum mothers; working with hard-to-reach populations; implementing problem-based learning for community health nursing courses; and offering multidisciplinary experiences for health professional trainees.
2. Community health centers and community development
a. Community health centers are ambulatory care outlets with a single point of access for patients, a coordinated multidisciplinary team, and multifunctional and community-oriented services.
b. These centers do not rely on fee-for-service payments. Services are provided through provincial health insurance plans.
c. Community health centers provide coverage for residents in a geographical catchment area.
H. Intersection of hospital and community care
1. Accessible primary health care includes recognition of the intersection of hospital and community services.

2. Sources of care in the home include home visits by nurses from public health agencies and home care programs.
3. Services include:
a. Treatments (dressing changes, medication administration, home dialysis)
b. Assistance with activities of daily living
c. Support services
d. Rehabilitation and maintenance services (physical therapy, occupational therapy)
e. Respite care
I. Working toward health public policy—Notable achievements in Canadian public health policies include mandatory seatbelt and infant carseat legislation, gun control regulations, and smoking restriction and taxation.

TEACHING STRATEGIES

1. Invite foreign-born nurses to speak to the class. Ask the nurses to discuss the health care system in their country of origin. Ask them to explain similarities and differences in philosophy of care (health vs. medical), financing of care, and structure of the system. How is the U.S. system superior? How is it inferior? How does nursing education differ?
2. Discuss positive and negative attributes of both the Cuban and Canadian health care systems. Would a system such as either of these work in the United States? Why or why not?

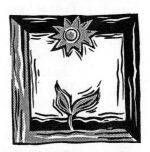

CHAPTER
30

Community Health Nursing: Making a Difference

ANNOTATED LEARNING OBJECTIVES

1. Discuss how being a member of an aggregate influences health.

People in a community share common characteristics. These characteristics can greatly affect the health of families and aggregates within that community. Shared characteristics of aggregates also aid in planning to meet the health needs. Some of these characteristics are socioeconomic status (individuals in lower socioeconomic groups have higher rates of morbidity and mortality than individuals in higher socioeconomic groups); gender (women have higher morbidity rates, and men have higher mortality rates); age (morbidity and mortality increase with age); race/ethnicity (partially attributed to inequality in income, education, and access to health care); social interaction (social support is a necessary factor in promoting heath and functional independence); and geography/politics.

2. Predict community health issues of the future based on shared characteristics of aggregates.

Changes in important community characteristics, such as socioeconomic status, gender, age, race and ethnicity, social interaction, and politics, will affect future health issues. Future health topics and health issues depend on several factors, including the aging of the U.S. population, increase in minority groups, increase in the number of people who are poor, and a variety of social problems.

Based on current trends, probable future health topics and health issues include AIDS and HIV infection; violence issues (abusive families, teenage gangs, use of illegal substances, increasing homicides, and suicides); health care for the elderly; Alzheimer's disease; equal access to health care for all; and funding of health care.

3. Describe actions needed by community health nurses to ensure future trends and changes in the health care system that will benefit the consumer of health care.

To address future needs and changes in the health care system, community health nurses should continue to work to expand scope of practice, particularly in independent nursing care for delivery of a wider variety of services to underserved aggregates. Nurses should focus on geriatric health needs; health care of minorities, with emphasis on cultural sensitivity; and use of the nursing process to care for aggregates and populations. Health promotion and illness prevention efforts should be expanded, and nurses must become involved in public policy issues related to health care. Finally, more research on aggregate health care and community health nursing issues should be encouraged.

LECTURE OUTLINE

I. **Community Characteristics That Affect Health**—Nurses have long been concerned with prevention and health promotion activities with individual patients, their families, and groups. Community health nursing extends nursing action to social units at the community, aggregate, and population levels. Shared characteristics are common to many people in the community. These characteristics will affect the health of families and communities and are important in determining their needs. Shared characteristics of aggregates also aid in planning to meet the health needs.

A. Socioeconomic status

1. Health is affected by socioeconomic status in that individuals in lower socioeconomic groups have higher rates of morbidity and

mortality than individuals in higher socio-economic groups.
2. Life expectancy is reduced by poverty through increased infant mortality, developmental limitations, chronic disease, and traumatic death. Infectious diseases, including HIV infection, are more common among those of lower socioeconomic status.

B. Gender
1. Gender affects health.
2. Women have higher morbidity rates, and men have higher mortality rates.
3. There is a gap of almost 7 years in life expectancy, with women living longer.

C. Age
1. Age is a very important determinant of health and is closely linked to morbidity and mortality.
2. More than 38% of people age 65+ have at least one limitation in activity.
   a. The primary needs of these individuals are for distributive, continuous care in the form of health monitoring, supervision, and periodic home health services.
   b. The health and surveillance needs of elders will continue to grow in the future.

D. Race and ethnicity—Health differences by race and ethnicity are partially attributed to inequality in income, education, and access to health care.

E. Social interaction
1. Relationships are important to health.
2. Social support is a necessary factor in promoting heath and functional independence.
3. Retirement, the loss of a spouse or close friend, and change in social contact are risk factors for disease and functional independence.
4. Factors such as role modeling and support from friends are important in health promotion.
5. Families influence personal health habits and physical environment.

F. Geography and politics—Political factors impact the delivery of health services at all levels. For example, Medicaid availability varies from state to state; as a consequence, health care for the poor varies simultaneously.

II. The Future of Public Health: What Are the Views of Public Health Nurses?
A. Several problems have been identified that demand aggregate action. These problems need to be addressed by community/public health nurses.

1. AIDS
2. Health care for the indigent
3. Injuries
4. Teen pregnancy
5. Hypertension
6. Smoking
7. Substance abuse
8. Hazardous waste
9. Alzheimer's disease

B. Greater representation by both women and nurses on policy-making boards can contribute positively to changes in public policy and aggregate interventions to address these needs.

III. Collective Activity for Health
A. Shared characteristics of aggregates that affect health are known as "risk factors" because they place an aggregate at risk.
B. Risk factors are key to community health nursing because they form the basis for assessment, planning, intervention, and evaluation.
C. Use of the nursing process at the aggregate level promotes changes based on characteristics of the aggregate.
D. These activities require community organization that involves planning and political activity by aggregates within the community.

IV. Determinants of Health
A. Research shows that individual, social, and environmental factors, rather than medical care, are the real determinants of health and that intervention at these levels is possible and makes a difference.
B. Consumers need to become more educated regarding the determinants of health beyond that of medical care.

V. Confusion Regarding Health, Health Care, and Medical Care
A. Health is usually viewed as a continuum from illness to peak potential.
B. Health is fluid.
1. Health changes in accordance with the goals and potential of aggregates within an environment.
2. It is affected by social units.
C. Medical care falls short of addressing the whole because it fails to address the complexity of factors that determine health.
1. The focus of medical care is typically on diagnosis and treatment of disease.
2. Medical care is necessary, but it has become too complex and highly specialized.
D. Health care of the individual, family, community, and society promotes self-care, medical

care, education, and political and environmental action.

E. The focus in health care is on the promotion of health and prevention of disease.

VI. Health As a Right

A. Health is viewed as a right, not a privilege; yet the major indicators of health in the United States are far below those of many other western countries.

B. Health must be defined by indigenous groups, the community, and society, and not by the outside professional.

C. Health care must not be confused with medical care, which is seen as a privilege and is experienced only by those who can afford it.
   1. Medical care is not a right in the United States.
   2. Funds in the United States go to medical care rather than to prevention and promotion, possibly because medical care generates revenue.

D. Health promotion and prevention cut back on the need for the largest U.S. industry: medical care.

E. For health care to be effective, there must be a sense of shared interest and community.

F. Health care professionals and consumers must work together to determine appropriate goals for health care and institute broad public health measures to prevent and decrease morbidity.

VII. Future Directions

A. The growing number of elders, homeless and disenfranchised, and uninsured must be addressed.

B. In general, Americans are in favor of universal coverage for health care and improving the efficiency of the health care industry.

C. Changes in reimbursement patterns and recognition of the benefits of providing preventive and supportive services in the community have driven changes in care delivery and will continue to cause change. Goals include:
   1. Achieving acceptable quality outcomes at acceptable costs
   2. Using professional resources as effectively and efficiently as possible
   3. Providing services in the most appropriate setting for the least cost
   4. Finding financial and other incentives for all concerned to work toward common goals

D. In the future, community health nurses may be caring for people on the basis of one of several

different models that promote community-based, aggregate care from a health promotion and wellness perspective.

VIII. Policy Implications

A. With the growth of capitation reimbursement, there is incentive to move services from institutions into the community.

B. Many organizations have not yet shifted to incorporation of prevention programs, using community health nurses as care providers, and creating services to match need.

C. Federal policy to promote these changes should be encouraged.

IX. Educational Implications

A. Today, more than ever, community heath nurses can make a difference.

B. Groups and aggregates cared for in the community now require a broad range of nursing services.

C. Fiscal realities and social demands mandate the continued growth of community-based care for the future.

D. Health educational systems must take action to prepare practitioners who are equipped to care for community's health by promoting healthy lifestyles and environments.

E. A change in nursing education to ensure that all nurses are prepared to function in a community-based health care system was posited by the NLN in 1993. To do this, nursing education programs must:
   a. Increase knowledge and practice of population-focused nursing
   b. Increase diversity of community health nursing students and practitioners
   c. Encourage community health nursing centers to provide accessible, prevention-oriented primary care
   d. Increase community organization, advocacy, and political activity.

TEACHING STRATEGIES

1. Obtain a copy of *Nursing's Agenda for Health Care Reform* and present excerpts to students. Have students debate the potential of the *Agenda* for addressing the health needs of at-risk populations. Discuss the necessity of policy changes to support reform.

2. Invite a guest from the local chapter of the American Nurses Association to speak about public policy issues related to nursing and health care. Ask the speaker to describe how can nurses become involved to cause changes in the health care system.

Calculation of Morbidity
and Mortality Rates

Calculation of Morbidity and Mortality Rates

Rates are used to facilitate interpretation of raw data and for comparisons. Rates are proportions or fractions in which the numerator is the number of events occurring in a specified period of time. Listed below are commonly used rates and calculation formulas.

For each rate listed below, "k" is an assigned value of 1000 or 100,000. The value of k is assigned so that the smallest rate calculated has at least one digit to the left of the decimal point (8.2/1000 rather than .82/10,000 and 8.5/100,000 rather than .85/1,000,000).

Incidence rates describe the occurrence of *new* disease cases in a community over a period of time relative to the size of the population at risk.

$$\text{Incidence rate} = \frac{\text{Number of } new \text{ cases during a specified period}}{\text{Population at risk during the same period}} \times k$$

Prevalence rates are the number of *all* cases of a specific disease in a population *at a given point in time* relative to the population at risk.

$$\text{Prevalence rate} = \frac{\text{Number of } existing \text{ cases at a specified time}}{\text{Population at risk at the same specific time}} \times k$$

Crude rates summarize the occurrence of births (crude birth rate) or deaths (crude death rate). The numerator is the number of events, and the denominator is the average population size.

$$\text{Crude death rate} = \frac{\text{Number of deaths in a population during a specified time}}{\text{Population estimate during the specified time}} \times k$$

$$\text{Crude birth rate} = \frac{\text{Number of live births during a specified time}}{\text{Population estimate during the specified time}} \times k$$

Specific rates are used to overcome some of the biases seen with crude rates. They are used to control for variables such as age, race, gender, and disease.

$$\text{Age-specific death rate} = \frac{\text{Number of deaths for a specified age group during a specified time}}{\text{Population estimate for the specified age group}} \times k$$

$$\text{Cause-specific death rate} = \frac{\text{Number of deaths from a specific cause during a specified time}}{\text{Population estimate during that time}} \times k$$

Exercise Problems for Calculation of Rates

Thirty-five new cases of tuberculosis were diagnosed in Utopia between January 1 and June 30, 1997. There were a total of 350 cases on the list of active cases at that same date (June 30). The population of Utopia as of March 30, 1997 was 250,000. Ten deaths had been attributed to tuberculosis during the first 6 months of 1997.

1. What is the incidence rate per 100,000 population for tuberculosis during that period?

2. What is the prevalence rate of tuberculosis per 100,000 on June 1, 1997?

3. What is the cause-specific death rate per 100,000 for tuberculosis?

During 1996, 215 new cases of were AIDS reported in Parkland, a city of 500,000. This brought the total number of active cases of AIDS to 2280. During that time, there were 105 deaths attributable to the disease.

4. What was the incidence rate per 100,000 for AIDS during 1996?

5. What was the prevalence rate of AIDS per 100,000?

6. What is the cause-specific death rate of AIDS?

Acme is a small city with a mid-1991 population of 120,000. During 1996, there were 342 live births and 515 deaths in Acme. Acme has a fairly large elderly population with approximately 24,000 of the population being over age 65. Of the 515 deaths during 1996, 425 were in individuals over 65.

7. What is the crude birth rate for Acme for 1996 per 1000?

8. What is the crude death rate for Acme for 1996 per 1000?

9. What is the age-specific death rate for individuals over age 65 for Acme for 1996 per 1000?

Answers to Exercises

1. $^{35}/_{250,000} \times 100,000 = 14$ cases per 100,000

2. $^{350}/_{250,000} \times 100,000 = 140$ cases per 100,000

3. $^{10}/_{250,000} \times 100,000 = 4$ deaths per 100,000

4. $^{215}/_{500,000} \times 100,000 = 43$ cases per 100,000

5. $^{2280}/_{500,000} \times 100,000 = 456$ cases per 100,000

6. $^{105}/_{500,000} \times 100,000 = 21$ deaths per 100,000

7. $^{342}/_{120,000} \times 1000 = 2.85$ births per 1000

8. $^{515}/_{120,000} \times 1000 = 4.29$ deaths per 1000

9. $425/_{24,000} \times 1000 = 17.71$ deaths over age 65 per 1000

Community Assessment Tool

Community Assessment Tool

I. Geography
   A. Topography
      1. Outline boundaries, examine and describe general physical features of the community.
      2. Identify physical features that might have an impact on health or health care delivery.
   B. Climate
      1. Describe climactic factors that might affect health and well-being.
      2. Describe existing efforts to manage those factors in at-risk populations (i.e., community efforts to pay heating bills for elders; shelter efforts to house the homeless during freezing weather; disaster relief plans).

II. Population
   A. Size—What is the total population of the community?
   B. Demographic characteristics
      1. Gender ratio—Are there more males or females, or are they evenly distributed?
      2. Age distribution—Is there a high percentage of small children? Elders?
      3. Race/ethnicity distribution—Describe percentages of primary racial/ethnic groups in the community.
   C. Trends
      1. Describe population changes in the community.
         a. During the past year
         b. During the past 5 years
         c. During the past 10 years
         d. During the past 20 years
      2. Outline anticipated changes over the next decade.
   D. Migration—Identify patterns or sources of migration or mobility.
      1. From what other areas do most residents move to this area?
      2. Where do they go when they leave?
      3. How long have most residents lived in the area?
   E. Density
      1. List the number of people per household.
      2. Identify and describe multiple-generation households.

III. Environment
   A. Water
      1. Identify the source of water for the area.
      2. Describe the water treatment process used.
   B. Sewage and waste disposal
      1. Identify the agency responsible for sewage disposal.
      2. Identify the agency responsible for waste disposal.
      3. Describe obvious, external sanitation problems.
         a. Is garbage collected regularly?
         b. Is trash evident on the streets and in vacant lots?
         c. Are abandoned cars or appliances in evidence?
   C. Air quality
      1. Identify the agency responsible for monitoring and maintaining clean air.
      2. Describe the most common threats to air quality.
      3. Identify measures that have been taken to alleviate threats to air quality.
   D. Food quality
      1. Identify the agency responsible for monitoring food quality and describe the process.
      2. What measures are taken when substandard food handling cases are identified? (For example, does the health department close down restaurants or grocery stores?

E. Housing
   1. Describe housing characteristics.
      a. Single- or multiple-family dwellings
      b. Number of rooms
      c. Number of bathrooms
      d. Average rent
   2. Observe and describe homes in the area.
      a. Of what materials are the homes constructed (frame, brick, etc.)?
      b. Are the homes well-kept?
      c. Are they air-conditioned?
      d. Are any broken windows evident?
      e. Do the homes need paint?
      f. Do they have burglar bars on the windows?
F. Animal control
   1. Observe for unleashed, unattended domestic animals. Are dogs and cats running loose?
   2. Are there any wild animals in the area that might pose a health threat? (skunks or raccoons with rabies, etc.)
   3. What agency is responsible for removing dead animals or catching unleashed dogs or cats?

IV. **Industry**
   A. Employment levels—Outline employment levels in the community.
   B. Manufacturing
      1. Identify major employers in the area.
      2. Does the community have large manufacturing plants?
         a. Are there any potential health threats related to employment in the plants?
         b. Is there any threat from the plant itself?
   C. White-collar vs. blue-collar—Identify the types of occupations of most residents (professional, service, manufacturing, farming, etc.).
   D. Income levels
      1. What is the median family income?
      2. What is the per capita income?

V. **Education**
   A. Schools—Visit and describe area schools.
   B. Level of education—What level of education have residents achieved?
   C. Literacy rates—Describe the literacy rates of the residents.
   D. Special education—What are the educational opportunities for children with special needs?
   E. School health services—Describe the health services in the community schools.
   F. School lunch programs
      1. Identify the agency responsible for setting the quality and nutritional guidelines for school lunches.
      2. Are there free or reduced-fee breakfast and lunch programs for low-income students? What are the qualification requirements?
   G. Access to higher education—Identify convenient opportunities for higher education.

VI. **Recreation**
   A. Parks and playgrounds
      1. Describe area parks and playgrounds.
      2. Are they clean and well-maintained?
      3. What agency or organization is responsible for maintenance?
      4. Is equipment in good repair? (Are swings broken? Is paint peeling? Are basketball nets missing?)
      5. Are children playing unsupervised?
   B. Libraries
      1. Identify the nearest library.
      2. Does the library have convenient hours?
      3. Does the library have programs to encourage children to read and to encourage general literacy?

C. Public and private recreation
1. Describe publicly sponsored opportunities for recreation (swimming pools, museums, etc.).
2. Describe private opportunities for recreation (movie theaters, amusement parks, theme parks, etc.).

VII. Religion

A. Churches, synagogues—Describe the number and location of churches.
B. Denominations—What denominations are represented by churches in the area?
C. Community programs—Describe community programs offered by area churches.
D. Health-related programs—Describe health-related programs offered by area churches.

VIII. Communication

A. Newspapers—Identify primary newspapers read by area residents.
B. Neighborhood news—Describe informal patterns of news dissemination (i.e., notes on telephone poles, posters in store windows, bulletin boards).
C. Radio and television
1. Are there local radio and television stations?
2. Do the stations provide local news and public service information?
D. Telephone—Do most residents have telephone service in their homes?
E. Hotlines
1. Identify local/regional hotlines (rape, suicide, poisoning, etc.).
2. Describe how the numbers for the hotlines are disseminated.

IX. Transportation

A. Intercity and intracity
1. Describe public transportation in the area. Include information about fares and convenience.
2. Is transportation available on weekends?
3. Describe transportation available between cities (bus, train, air, etc.).
B. Handicapped services—Describe transportation services for the handicapped.
1. How are these services accessed?
2. What are the fees for the services?
C. Emergency transportation—Describe the available ambulance services.
1. Are the services professional or voluntary?
2. What are the average response times?
3. What are the fees for transport?

X. Public Services

A. Fire protection—Identify the nearest fire station. What are average response times?
B. Police protection—Identify the nearest police station.
1. What are average response times?
2. Is police presence evident in the community?
C. Rape treatment centers—Identify resources for rape treatment. How are these services accessed?
D. Utilities—Describe organizations responsible for providing public utilities.
1. Are utility services reliable?
2. Are they affordable?

XI. Political Organization

A. Structure—What is the structure of the local government?
B. Methods for filling positions—How are positions in local government filled?
C. Responsibilities of positions
1. What are the responsibilities of the main political figures?
2. Is someone responsible for the health of the community? If so, what are that person's responsibilities?
D. Sources of revenue—What are the main sources of revenue for public services?
E. Voter registration
1. What percentage of voters are registered?
2. What percentage of voters voted in the last local election?

XII. Community Development or Planning
   A. Activities—Identify current projects affecting health that are currently in progress.
   B. Major issues—Describe the major issues in community development and planning.

XIII. Disaster Programs
   A. American Red Cross
      1. Identify the closest chapter of the American Red Cross.
      2. What programs and services does the American Red Cross offer in the area?
   B. Potential sources of disaster—Identify potential sources of disasters (hurricanes, earthquakes, airline crashes, refinery fires, etc.).
   C. Disaster plans—Describe disaster plans outlined by local government.

XIV. Health Statistics
   A. Mortality
      1. Identify the leading causes of death in the area.
      2. List the number of deaths due to major causes (heart disease, cancer, CVA, HIV, etc.) by age and race/ethnic group.
   B. Morbidity—Describe the leading causes of morbidity in the area. Include information about reportable communicable diseases.
   C. Births
      1. List births by age and race/ethnic group.
      2. Identify the number of births with no or late prenatal care.
      3. Identify the number of births with low-birthweight infants and other negative outcomes.

XV. Social Problems
   A. Mental health
      1. Describe the rates of mental illness in the community.
      2. Are there any organized efforts to improve mental health?
   B. Alcoholism and drug abuse—Describe the impact of drug and alcohol use on the residents.
   C. Suicide
      1. Outline any suicides by age and race/ethnic group.
      2. Has there been any trend of increase or decrease in suicide rates?
   D. Crime
      1. Obtain crime statistics for the area.
      2. Describe the most common types of crime (violent crimes, theft and burglary, vandalism).
   E. School dropout rate
      1. Identify the percentage of residents who drop out of school each year.
      2. Describe the profile of dropouts (predominantly male, minority, etc.).
   F. Unemployment—Define unemployment levels in the area.
   G. Gangs
      1. Describe gang involvement in the area.
      2. Is there evidence of morbidity and mortality in the area due to gangs?
      3. Has there been related devaluation of property?

XVI. Health Manpower
   A. Obtain information about numbers of licensed health personnel (nurses, physicians, pharmacists, dentists, etc.) currently practicing in the area.
   B. Does the supply of primary health care providers appear to be adequate?

XVII. Community Services
   A. Institutional care—Describe numbers and types of institutional care facilities (hospitals, nursing homes).
   B. Ambulatory care—Describe numbers and types of ambulatory care facilities (clinics, doctor's offices).
   C. Preventive health services—Describe organizational and community-based efforts to provide preventive health care.
   D. Nursing services—Describe available nursing services.

Community Assessment Tool

Physical Environment

Community location (boundaries, urban/rural): _____
_____
_____

Size and density: _____
_____
_____

Prominent topographical features: _____
_____
_____

Housing *(type, conditions, adequacy, number of people per dwelling, sanitation):* _____
_____
_____
_____

Safety hazards present in the environment: _____
_____
_____

Source of community water supply: _____
_____
_____

Sewage and waste disposal: _____
_____
_____

Nuisance factors: _____
_____
_____

Psychological Environment

Future prospects for the community: _____
_____
_____

Significant events in community history: _____
_____
_____

Interaction of groups within the community *(racial tension, etc.):* _____
_____
_____

Protective services *(adequacy, local crime rate, insurance rates):* _____
_____
_____

Communication network *(media, informal channels, links to outside world):* _____
_____
_____

Sources of stress in the community: _____
_____
_____

Extent of mental illness in the community: _____
_____
_____

Social Environment
Government *(type effectiveness, officials):* _____
_____
_____

Unofficial leaders *(significant informants):* _____
_____
_____

Political affiliations of community members: _____
_____
_____

Status of minority groups *(influence, length of residence):* _____
_____
_____

Languages spoken by community members: _____
_____

Community income levels *(poverty, coverage by assistance programs):* _____
_____
_____

Education *(prevailing levels, attitudes, facilities):* _____
_____

Religion *(major affiliations, programs and services, influence on health):* _____
_____
_____

Culture *(affiliation, influence on health):* _____
_____
_____

Overhead Transparency Masters

Chapter 1
Health: A Social, Personal, and Political View

Characteristics of the U.S. Health Care System

Definitions of Health

Definitions of Public Health and Community Health

Preventive Approach to Health

Public and Community Health Nursing

Chapter 2
Historical Factors: Community Health Nursing in Context

Evolution of the State of Health of Western Populations

Hunting and Gathering Stage

Settled Village State

Preindustrial Cities Stage

Industrial Cities Stage

Present Stage

Evolution of Early Public Health Efforts

Prehistoric Times

Classical Times

Middle Ages

Renaissance

Eighteenth Century

Nineteenth Century

Advent of Modern Health Care

Community Caregiver

Establishment of Public Health Nursing

Consequences for the Health of Aggregates

Challenges for Community Health Nursing

Chapter 3
The Health Care System: United States

Major Legislation and the Health Care System

Pure Food and Drugs Act (1906)

Children's Bureau (1912)

Shepard-Towner Act (1921)

Hill-Burton Act (1946)

Department of Health, Education, and Welfare (1953)

Nurse Training Act (1964)

Social Security Act (1935, Amended in 1965 and 1972)

National Health Planning and Resources Act (1974)

Omnibus Budget Reconciliation Act (1981)

Social Security Act Amendment (1983)

Family Support Act (1988)

Health Objectives Act 2000 (1990)

Redefining Health

Components of the Health Care System

Roles of the Federal Government in Public Health

Roles of the State Government in Public Health

Roles of the Local Government in Public Health

Future of the Health Care System

Chapter 4
Thinking Upstream: Conceptualizing Health from a Population Perspective

Thinking Upstream: Looking Beyond the Individual

Historic Perspectives on Nursing Theory

Issues of Fit

Definitions of Theory

Theory to What End?

Microscopic vs. Macroscopic Approaches to the Conceptualization of Community Health Problems

Scope of Theory in Community Health Nursing

Microscopic Theories

Macroscopic Theories

Chapter 5
Community Assessment and Epidemiology

The Nature of a Community

Assessing the Community: Sources of Data

Census Data

Vital Statistics

Other Sources of Health Data

Assessing the Community: The Use of Rates

Epidemiology

Definition

Purpose

Epidemiological Triangle

Wheel Model

Web of Causation

Use in Secondary and Tertiary Prevention

Establishing Causality

Screening

Surveillance

Use in Health Services

(Continued on next page)

Chapter 5, continued

Types of Epidemiology

Descriptive Epidemiology

Analytic Epidemiology

Epidemiological Methods

Cross-Sectional (Prevalence or Correlational) Studies

Retrospective (Case Control) Studies

Prospective (Longitudinal or Cohort) Studies

Experimental Studies

Application of the Nursing Process

Chapter 6
Community Health
Planning and Evaluation

Overview of Health Planning

Health Planning Model

Assessment

Planning

Intervention

Evaluation

Health Planning Projects

Health Planning Legislation

Early Efforts

Hill-Burton Act (1946)

Heart Disease, Cancer, and Stroke Amendments (1965)

Public Health Service Act Amendments (1966)

Certificate of Need

National Health Planning and Resources Development Act (1974)

The 1980s

The 1990s

Nursing Implications

Chapter 7
Community Organization: Building Partnerships for Health

Conceptual Basis of Community Organization

Social Systems Theories

Social Change

Community Participation

Definition of Community Organization

Community Organization Models

Rothman's Community Organization Typology

Primary Health Care

Public Health Models and Frameworks

Community Organization of Nursing Care of Aggregates

Application of the Nursing Process Through Community Organization

Social Planning

Social Action

Community Development

Chapter 8
Community Health Education

Health Education in the Community

Learning Theories, Principles, and Health Education Models

Learning Theories

Knowles' Assumptions About Characteristics of Adult Learners

Health Education Models

Community Empowerment

The Nurse's Role in Health Education

Putting Models and Theories into Action

Stage I: Planning and Strategy Selection

Stage II: Selecting Channels and Materials

Stage III: Developing Materials and Pretesting

Stage IV: Implementation

Stage V: Assessing Effectiveness

Stage VI: Feedback to Refine Program

Health Education Resources

Chapter 9
Policy, Politics, Legislation, and Public Health Nursing

Nurses Who Made a Difference

Florence Nightingale

Carrie Long

Nurses: Agents of Change

Public Policy: Blueprint for Governance

Policy Formulation in an "Ideal World"

Policy Formulation in the "Real World"

Steps in Policy Formation

Policy Analysis

Health Care Reform and the Nursing Agenda

Government: The Hallmark of Civilization

Government Authority for the Protection of the Public's Health

Balance of Powers: Safeguard of Government

Politics in Action—The Legislative Process

The Individual Nurse's Role in Politics

The Collective Power of Nurses

Nursing and the Health of the Nation—A Social Contract

Chapter 10
Child and Adolescent Health

Indicators of Child and Adolescent Health Status

Pregnancy and Infancy

Infant Mortality

Low Birthweight

Lack of Prenatal Care

Prenatal Substance Use

Childhood

Accidental Injuries

Lead Poisoning

Child Abuse and Neglect

Adolescence

Violence

Teenage Pregnancy

Sexually Transmitted Diseases

Substance Abuse

Social Factors Affecting Child Health

Poverty

Single-Parent Households

Adolescence

(Continued on next page)

Chapter 10, continued

Costs to Society for Poor Health Among Children

Prenatal Care

Lead Poisoning

Adolescent Pregnancy and Parenting

Public Health Programs Targeted to Children

Medicaid

Maternal and Child Health Block Grants

Community and Migrant Health Centers Program

National Health Service Corps

Supplemental Food Program for Women, Infants, and Children (WIC)

Head Start

Strategies to Improve Child Health

Parent's Role

Community's Role

Employers' Role

Government's Role

Community Health Nurses' Role

Chapter 11
Women's Health

Major Indicators of Health

Life Expectancy

Mortality

Morbidity

Mental Health

Other Factors

Types of Problems

Acute Illness

Chronic Disease

Reproductive Health

Sexually Transmitted Diseases and HIV

Unintentional Injury (Accidents)

Disability

Major Legislation Affecting Women's Health Services

Public Health Service Act (1982)

Civil Rights Act (1964)

Social Security Act

Occupational Safety and Health Act

Family and Medical Leave Act (1993)

(Continued on next page)

Chapter 11, continued

Health and Social Services to Promote Women's Health

Roles of the Community Health Nurse

Research in Women's Health

Office of Research on Women's Health

Women's Health Initiative

Chapter 12
Men's Health

Traditional Indicators of Men's Health Status

Longevity

Mortality

Morbidity

Use of Medical Care

Theories That Explain Men's Health

Biological Factors

Socialization

Orientation Toward Illness and Prevention

Reporting Health Behavior

Interpreting Data

Factors That Impede Men's Health

Medical Care Patterns

Access to Care

Lack of Health Promotion

(Continued on next page)

Chapter 12, continued

Factors That Promote Men's Health

Interest Groups in Men's Health

Increasing Interest in Physical Fitness and Lifestyle

Policy Related to Men's Health

Health Services for Men

Men's Health Care Needs

Meeting Men's Health Needs

Application of the Nursing Process

Roles of the Community Health Nurse

Research and Men's Health

Web Resources on Men's Health

Chapter 13
Family Health

The Changing Family

Definition of the Family

Characteristics of the Changing Family

Approaches to Meeting the Health Needs of Families

Nursing in a Family Context

Moving from the Individual to the Family

Family Interviewing

Moving from the Family to the Community

Family Theory Approach to Meeting the Health Needs of Families

Reasons for Working with Families

Systems Approach

Structural-Functional Conceptual Framework

Assessment Tools

Genogram

Family Health Tree

Ecomap

Family Health Assessment

Social and Structural Constraints

(Continued on next page)

Chapter 13, continued

Extending Family Health Intervention to Larger Aggregates and Social Action

Institutional Context of Family Therapists

Models of Social Class and Health Services

Models of Care for Communities of Families

Application of the Nursing Process

The Home Visit

The Nursing Process in Home Health Care

Chapter 14
Senior Health

Major Indicators of Health in the Elderly

Definitions

Elderly Population in the United States

Mortality

Morbidity

Health Behavior and Health Care

Income

Literacy and Education

Marital Status, Relationships, and Living Arrangements

Religion

Problems of the Elderly

Difficulties at Home

Nutrition Needs

Disability

Accidents

Medications

Thermal Stress

Preventing Illness and Hospitalization

Hospitalization Issues

(Continued on next page)

Chapter 14, continued

Institutionalization

Death and Bereavement

Community Environment

Abuse of the Elderly

Crime and the Elderly

Families of the Elderly

Major Legislation for the Elderly

The Social Security Act

The Older Americans Act

Research on Aging Act

Age Discrimination in Employment Act

Employee Retirement Income Security Act

Retirement Equity Act

New Concepts of Community Care

Application of the Nursing Process

Allocation of Resources for Senior Health

Research on the Health of the Elderly

Roles of the Community Health Nurse

Chapter 15
The Homeless

Definitions and Prevalence of Homelessness

Factors That Contribute to Homelessness

Poverty

Changes in the Labor Market

Lack of Affordable Housing

Deinstitutionalization

Heavy Use of Alcohol and Illicit Drugs

Health State of the Homeless

Homeless Men

Homeless Women

Homeless Children

Homeless Adolescents

Homeless Families

Homeless People with Mental Health or Substance Use Problems

Health Care Access for the Homeless Population

Conceptual Approaches to Health Care for the Homeless Population

Application of the Nursing Process

Research and the Homeless

Chapter 16
Rural Health

Rural United States

Community and Statistical Indicators of Rural Health

Variation in Rural Communities

Barriers to Health Care

Structural, Financial, and Personal Factors and Health Status

Specific Rural Aggregates: Agricultural Workers

Impact of Agriculture on Rural Health

Accidents and Injuries

Acute and Chronic Illnesses

Migrant and Seasonal Farm Workers

Application of Theories and "Thinking Upstream" Concepts to Rural Health

Attach Community-Based Problems at Their Roots

Emphasize the "Doing" Aspects of Health

Maximize the Use of Informal Networks

Rural Health Care Delivery System

Rural Health Care Statistics

Alternative Facility Model

(Continued on next page)

Chapter 16, continued

   Health Care Provider Shortages

   Community-Wide Health Care System

   Primary Care and Primary Health Care

Community-Based Care

   Home Care and Hospice Programs

   Rural Mental Health Care

   Emergency Services

   Informal Care Systems

   Rural Public Health Departments

   Managed Care in the Rural Environment

Legislation and Programs Affecting Public Health

Rural Community Health Nursing

Application of the Nursing Process

Rural Health Research

Chapter 17
Sociocultural Diversity and Community Health Nursing

Transcultural Perspectives on Community Health Nursing

Population Trends

Historical Perspective on Cultural Diversity

Transcultural Nursing in the Community

Definition and Origin

Culture in Transcultural Nursing

Formation of Values

Family

Socioeconomic Factors

Socioeconomic Status

Distribution of Resources

Education

Culture and Nutrition

Culture and Religion

Cross-Cultural Communication

Cultural Background

Definition of Cross-Cultural Communication

(Continued on next page)

Chapter 17, continued

Space, Distance, and Intimacy

Overcoming Communication Barriers

Nonverbal Communication

Touch

Sex

Language

Health-Related Beliefs and Practices

Health, Illness, and Cultural Diversity

Cultural Expression of Illness

Culture and Treatment

Cultural Negotiation

Solutions to Health Care Problems in Culturally Diverse Populations

Role of the Community Health Nurse in Improving Health for Culturally Diverse People

Research Agenda

Chapter 18
Cultural Influence in the Community: The African-American Community

African-American History

African-Americans in Contemporary Society

Social Justice: An African-American Perspective

  Self-Concept, Racism, and Racial Identity

  Profiles of African-Americans

  Racism

  African-American Cultural Beliefs

  African-American World View and Cultural Precepts

  Changing Patterns of African-American Family Life

  Gender Roles

Communication and Language

Health Beliefs and Practices

  Traditional Beliefs About Health and Illness

  Sociopolitical Variations in Health and Illness

  Indicators of Health in the African-American Population

  Alcohol Problems

  Drug-Related Problems

  Homicide and Unintentional Injuries

(Continued on next page)

Chapter 18, continued

Nursing Care of African-Americans

Cultural Sensitivity

Chapter 19
Cultural Influence in the Community: The Mexican-American Community

Understanding Mexican-American Health Needs

Disease Prevalence in the Mexican-American Community and Access to Health Care

The Mexican-American Family

Traditional Mexican-American Families

Nontraditional Mexican-American Families

Beliefs of Disease Causation Among Mexican-Americans

Health and Disease

Folk Healing

Diseases Caused by Dislocation of Internal Organs

Diseases of Emotional Origin

Disease of Magical Origin—*Mal Ojo*

The Hot-Cold Syndrome

Use of Herbal Medicine

Cultural Adaptation to Health Care

Improving Health Education and Communication

Chapter 21
Violence in the Community

History of Abuse

Scope of the Problem

Homicide

Suicide

Assault

Impact of Guns

Violence of Aggregates

Youth-Related Violence

Domestic Violence

Child Abuse

Abuse of the Elderly

Public Health Perspective

Prevention of Violence in the Community

Safety of the Health Professional

Nursing Diagnoses for Victims of Abuse

Chapter 22
Mental Health

Mental Health

Community Mental Health Movement

Characteristics of Community Mental Health

The Three Phases of Psychiatric Evolution

Legislation

Factors Contributing to the Mental Health of Aggregates

Environmental Factors

Biological Factors

Social Factors

Assessment of Aggregate Mental Health

Nursing Process

Roles of the Community Mental Health Nurse

Phases of the Therapeutic Relationship

Application of the Nursing Process to Community Mental Health

Chapter 23
Substance Abuse in the Community

Historic Trends in the Use of Alcohol and Illicit Drugs

Prevalence of Substance Abuse

Concepts of Substance Abuse

Definitions

Cause of Substance Abuse

Sociocultural and Political Aspects of Substance Abuse

Crack Cocaine Epidemic

Typical Course of Addictive Illness

Modes of Intervention

Overview

Treatment

Pharmacotherapies

Issues Unique to Substance Abuse

Relapse Prevention

Mutual Help Groups

Social Network Involvement

Family and Friends

Effects on the Family

Professional Enablers

(Continued on next page)

Chapter 23, continued

Vulnerable Aggregates

Adolescents

Elderly

Women

Minority Groups

Other Aggregates

Nursing Perspective on Substance Abuse

Nursing Interventions in the Community

Chapter 24
Communicable Disease

The Communicable Disease Spectrum

Transmission

Direct Transmission

Indirect Transmission

Fecal-Oral Transmission

Airborne Transmission

Immunity

Prevention

Universal Blood and Body Fluid Precautions

Defining and Reporting Cases

Control

Elimination

Eradication

Vaccine-Preventable Diseases

Recommended Vaccine Schedules

Vaccines

Types of Immunization

Vaccine Storage, Transport, and Handling

(Continued on next page)

Chapter 24, continued

Vaccine Administration and Routes

Vaccine Dosages

Vaccine Spacing

Vaccine Hypersensitivity

Vaccine Documentation

Reporting Adverse Events

Vaccine Needs for Special Groups

Adolescents and Young Adults

Adults and Elders

Immunosuppression

Pregnancy

Vaccine-Preventable Diseases

Diphtheria

Haemophilus Influenza Type B (Hib)

Hepatitis A and B

Influenza Types A, B, and C

Measles

Mumps

Pertussis

Polio

Rubella

(Continued on next page)

Chapter 24, continued

Tetanus

Varicella

Vaccines for International Travel

Cholera

Japanese Encephalitis

Meningococcus

Plague

Rabies

Tuberculosis

Typhoid

Yellow Fever

Sexually Transmitted Diseases

AIDS/HIV

Chlamydia

Gonorrhea

Herpes Simplex Virus 2

Human Papillomavirus

Syphilis

Prevention of Communicable Diseases

Chapter 25
School Health

A Critical Theory Approach to School Health

The Context of School Health

Indicators of School Health Status

Components of a School Health Program

School Health Services

School Health Education

School Health Environment

Additional Components of a Comprehensive School Health Program

School Health Financing

School Health Delivery Models

The Practice of Nursing in the Schools

Levels of Prevention

Nursing Process

Research in School Health

Chapter 26
Environmental Health

A Critical Theory Approach to Environmental Health

Areas of Environmental Health

Living Patterns

Work Risks

Atmospheric Quality

Water Quality

Housing

Food Quality

Waste Control

Radiation Risks

Violence Risks

Effects of Environmental Hazards

Efforts to Control Environmental Health Problems

Approaching Environmental Health at the Aggregate Level

Critical Community Health Nursing Practice

Chapter 27
Occupational Health

Definition of Occupational Health Nursing

Evolution of Occupational Health Nursing

Roles of the Occupational Health Nurse

Demographic Trends and Effects on Occupational Health Nursing

Demographic Trends That Affect Occupational Health Nursing

Increased Emphasis on Roles in Prevention

Women in the Workplace

Minorities in the Workplace

Delivery and Access Issues Related to Health Care

AIDS in the Workplace

AAOHN Year 2000 Recommendations

Skills and Competencies of the Occupational Health Nurse

Management and Administration

Direct Care

Health and Environmental Relationships

Legal and Ethical Responsibilities

Consultation

(Continued on next page)

Chapter 27, continued

Research

Health Education

Counseling

Primary, Secondary, and Tertiary Levels of Prevention

The Impact of Legislation on Occupational Health

The Occupational Safety and Health Act (1970)

Workers' Compensation Acts

The Americans with Disabilities Act (1991)

Professional Liability

Multidisciplinary Teamwork

Chapter 28
The Home Visit and Home Health Care

Home Health Care

Purpose of Home Health Services

Conducting a Home Visit Using the Nursing Process

Visit Preparation

Referral

Initial Telephone Contact

Environment

Safety Issues

Building Trust

Application of the Nursing Process

Types of Home Health Agencies

Official Agencies

Nonprofit Agencies

Proprietary Agencies

Chains

Hospital-Based Agencies

Certified and Noncertified Agencies

Special Home Health Programs

Reimbursement for Home Care

(Continued on next page)

Chapter 28, continued

Educational Preparation of Home Health Nurses

Documentation of Home Care

The Family or Caregiver in Home Care

Hospice Home Care

Characteristics of Hospice Home Care

Caring for the Caregiver

Pain Control and Symptom Management

Chapter 29
World Health

Population Growth

Environmental Stressors

Types of Environmental Stressors

Patterns of Disease

Promoting Health in Developing Countries

Promoting Health in Developed Countries

Primary Health Care in Cuba

World Health Organization's Definition of Primary Health Care

History of the Development of Cuba's Primary Health Care Model

Cuba's Neighborhood/Home Clinics

Achievements in Health As a Result of Cuba's Model for Women's Health

Consequences of Cuba's Model for Women's Health

Effects of Economic Hardships on Cuba's Health Care Model

Critique of Cuba's Model

Primary Health Care in Canada

Characteristics of Canadian Health Care

Emergence of a Universal Health Care System

Changing Paradigms for Health Care Delivery

(Continued on next page)

Chapter 29, continued

Rising Cost of Health Care

Transitions in Community Health Nursing

New Roles for the Community Health Nurse in Canada

Innovative Health Care Delivery Models

Intersection of Hospital and Community Care

Chapter 30
Community Health Nursing: Making a Difference

Community Characteristics That Affect Health

Socioeconomic Status

Gender

Age

Race and Ethnicity

Social Interaction

Geography and Politics

The Future of Public Health

Collective Activity for Health

Determinants of Health

Confusing Regarding Health, Health Care, and Medical Care

Health As a Right

Future Directions

Policy Implications

Educational Implications

Figure 1–1
The Three Levels of Prevention

Level 1. **Primary Prevention Activities**

Prevention of problems before they occur

Example: Immunizations

Level 2. **Secondary Prevention Activities**

Early detection and intervention

Example: Screening for sexually transmitted disease

Level 3. **Tertiary Prevention Activities**

Correction and prevention of deterioration of a disease state

Example: Teaching insulin administration in the home

Figure 2–1
Stages in the Disease History of Humankind

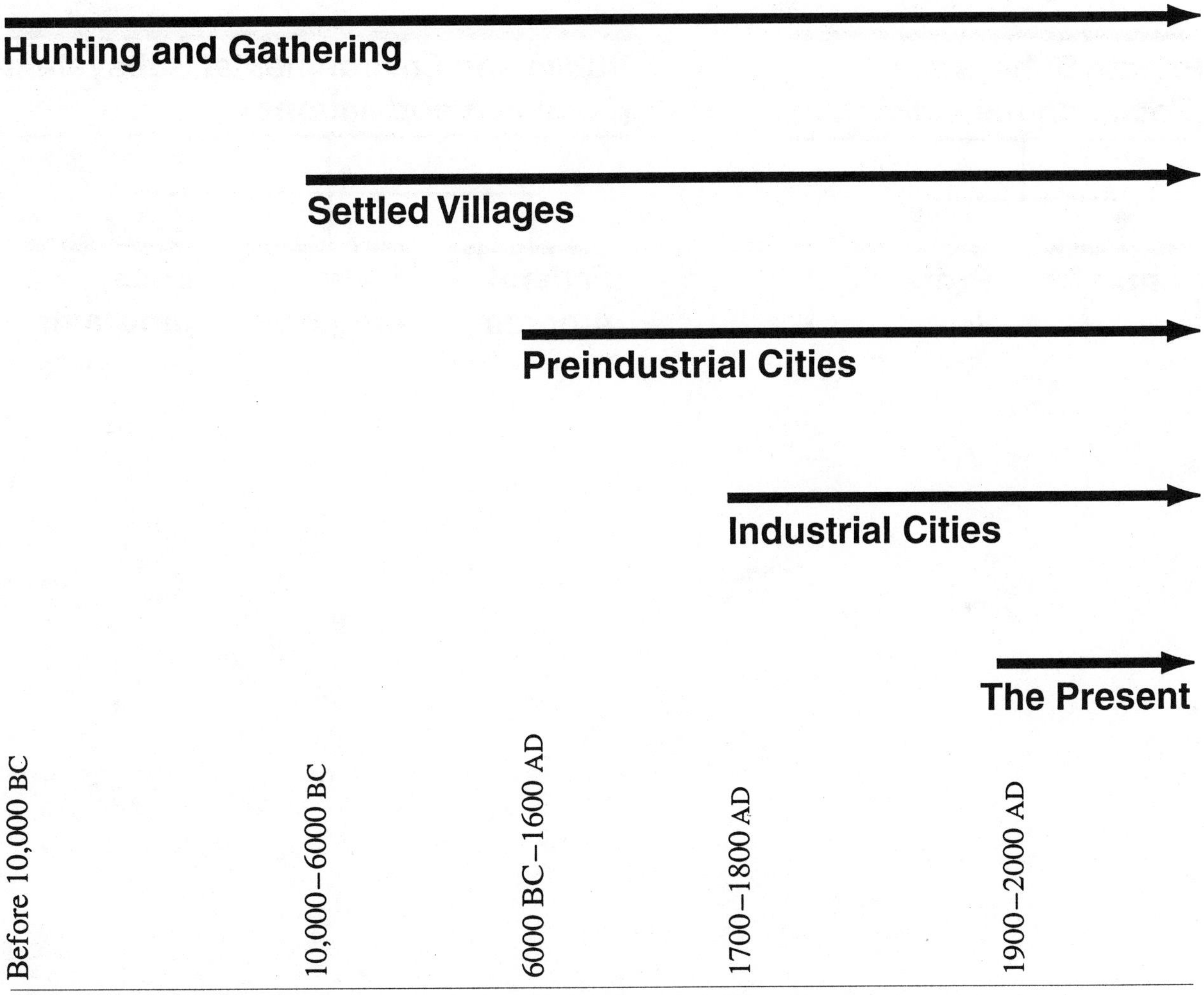

Hunting and Gathering →

Settled Villages →

Preindustrial Cities →

Industrial Cities →

The Present →

Before 10,000 BC

10,000–6000 BC

6000 BC–1600 AD

1700–1800 AD

1900–2000 AD

Stages overlap and time periods are widely debated in the field of anthropology. Some form of each stage remains evident in the world today.

Figure 3–1
U.S. Health Care System

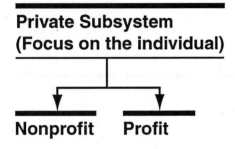

**Private Subsystem
(Focus on the individual)**

Nonprofit   Profit

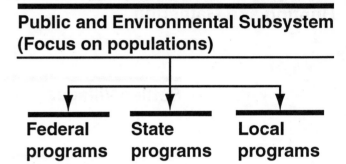

**Public and Environmental Subsystem
(Focus on populations)**

Federal   State   Local
programs   programs   programs

Figure 5–1
Prevalence Pot: The Relationship Between Incidence and Prevalence

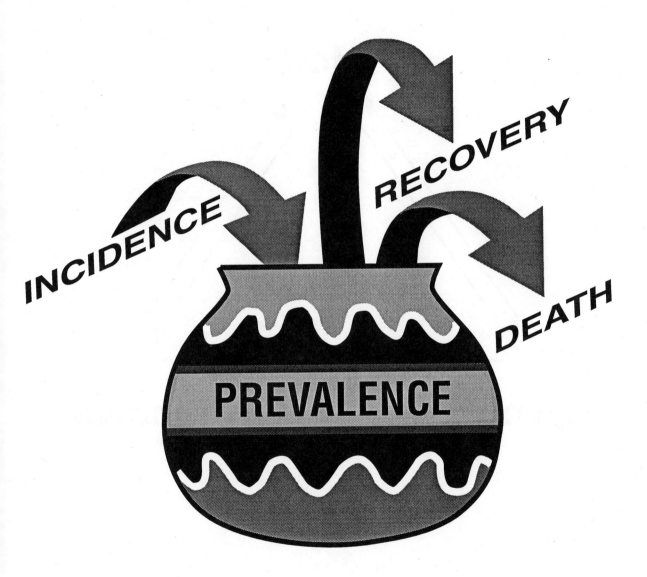

Redrawn from Morton RF, Hebel JR, McCarter RJ: A Study Guide to Epidemiology and Biostatistics, 3rd ed. Gaithersburg, MD: Aspen Publishers, 1990, p. 30. Copyright © 1990 by Aspen Publishers, Inc.

Figure 5–2
Epidemiological Triangle

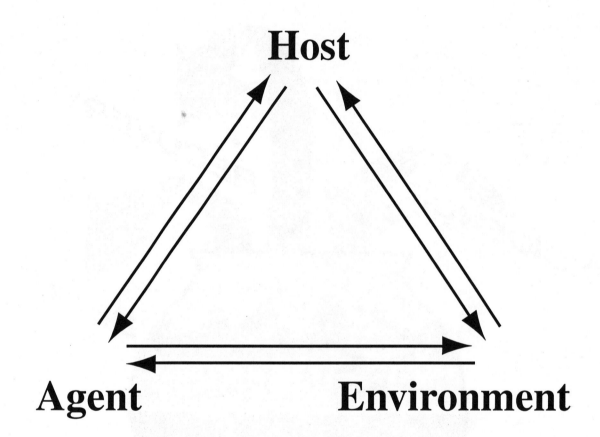

Figure 5–3
Wheel Model of Human-Environment Interaction

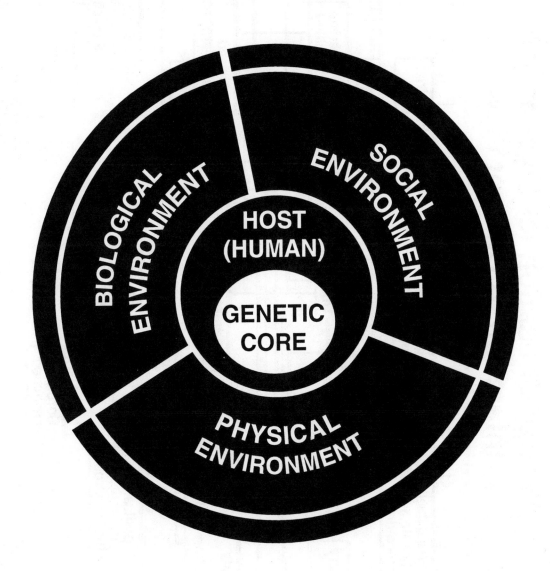

Redrawn from Mausner, JS, Kramer, S: Mausner and Bahn Epidemiology: An Introductory Text, 2nd ed. Philadelphia: WB Saunders, 1985, p. 36.

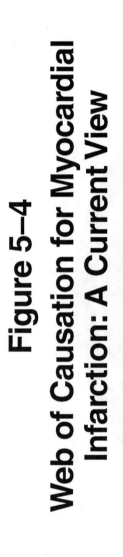

Figure 5–4

Web of Causation for Myocardial Infarction: A Current View

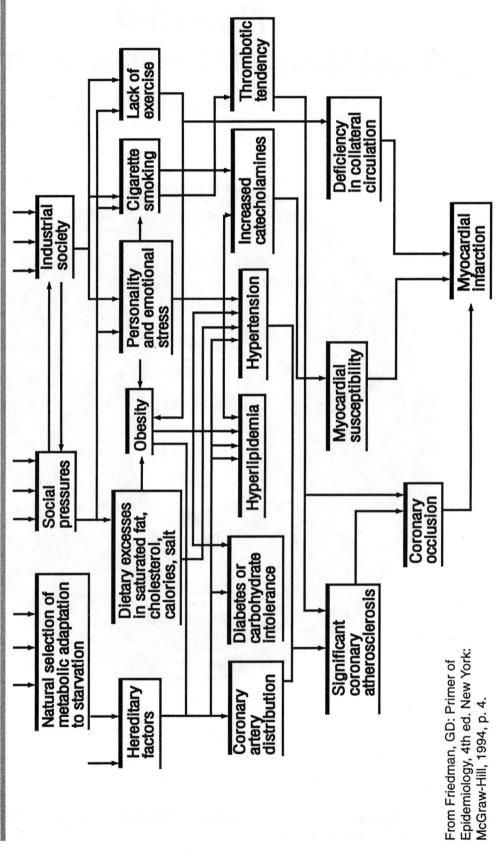

From Friedman, GD: Primer of Epidemiology, 4th ed. New York: McGraw-Hill, 1994, p. 4.

Figure 5–9
Format for Community Health Diagnosis

Increased risk of _____
(disability, disease, etc.)

among _____ **related to**
(community or population)

_____ **as demonstrated**
(etiological statement)

in _____ .
(health indicators)

Redrawn from Muecke MA: Community health diagnosis in nursing. Pub Health Nurs *1;*23, 1984. Used with permission of Blackwell Scientific Publications.

Figure 6–1
The Community As Client

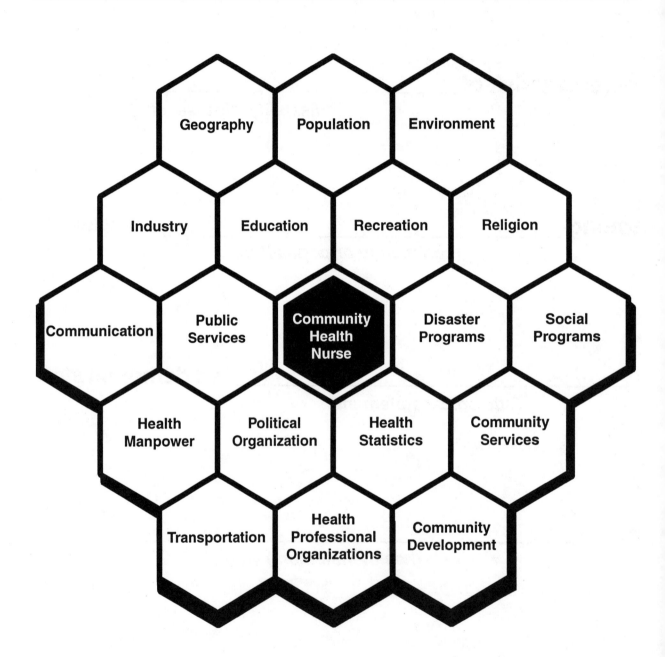

Figure 6–2
Health Planning Model

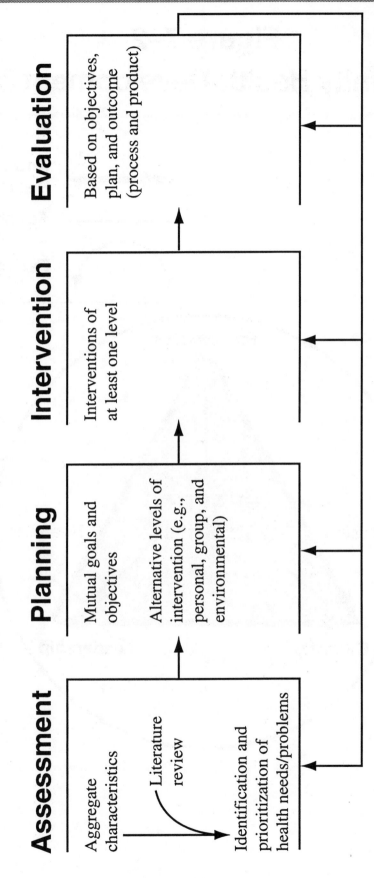

Figure 7–2
Community Health Development Model

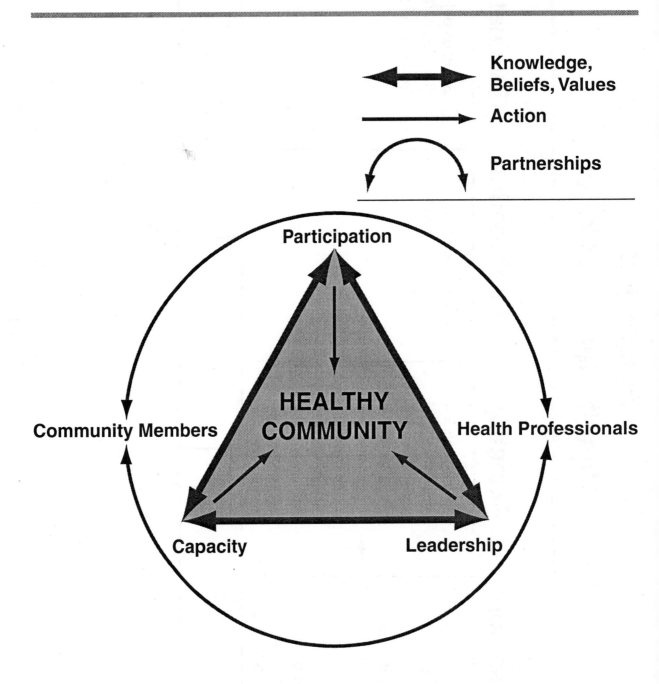

Figure 8–1
Framework for Developing Health Communications

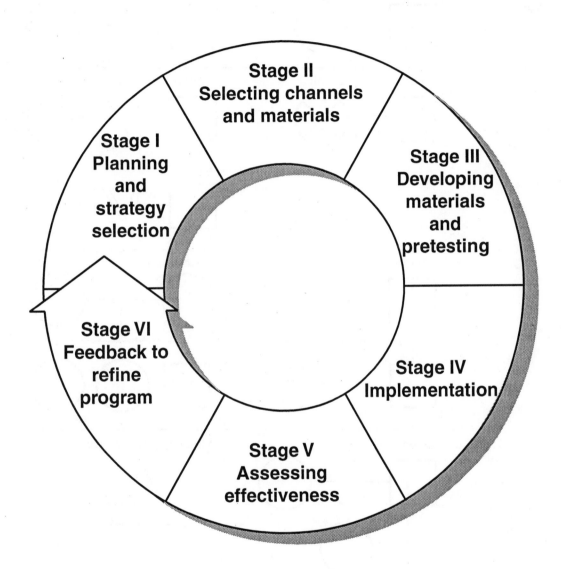

The National Cancer Institute suggests using this model to develop health education messages. (Data from U.S. Department of Health and Human Services, 1992.)

Figure 13–2
Genogram and Attachment Symbols

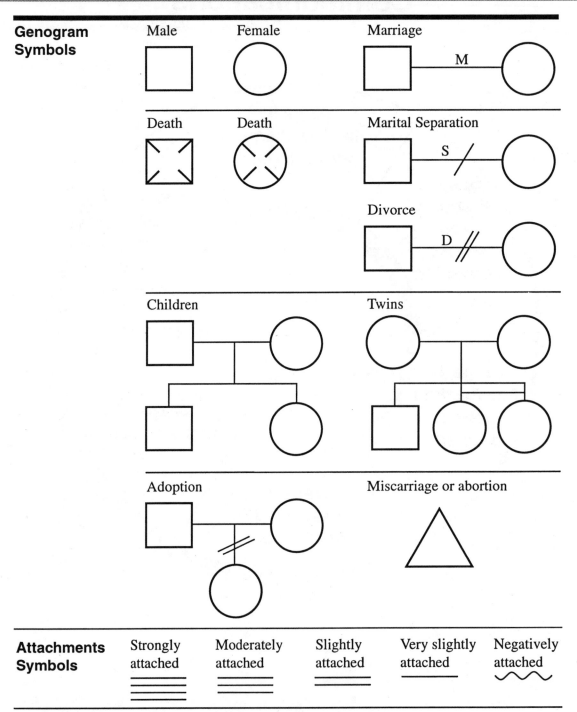

Genogram Symbols

Male | Female | Marriage — M

Death | Death | Marital Separation — S

Divorce — D

Children | Twins

Adoption | Miscarriage or abortion

Attachments Symbols

Strongly attached | Moderately attached | Slightly attached | Very slightly attached | Negatively attached

Redrawn from Wright, L.M., and Leahey, M.: Nurses and Families: A Guide to Family Assessment and Intervention. Philadelphia: F.A. Davis, 1984.

Figure 13–4
Chan Family Health Tree

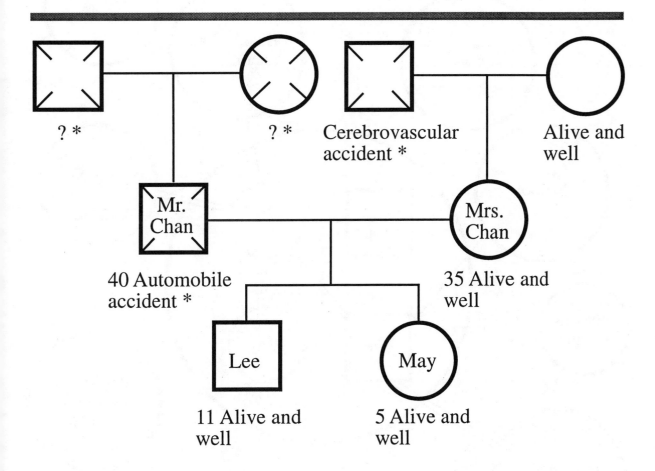

? *   ? *   Cerebrovascular   Alive and
                                      accident *   well

Mr.   Mrs.
Chan   Chan

40 Automobile   35 Alive and
accident *   well

        Lee   May

11 Alive and   5 Alive and
well   well

Modified from Diekelman, N.: Primary Health Care of the Well Adult. New York, McGraw-Hill, 1977.
Reproduced with permission of McGraw-Hill, Inc.

Figure 13–6
Sample Ecomap of Chan Family

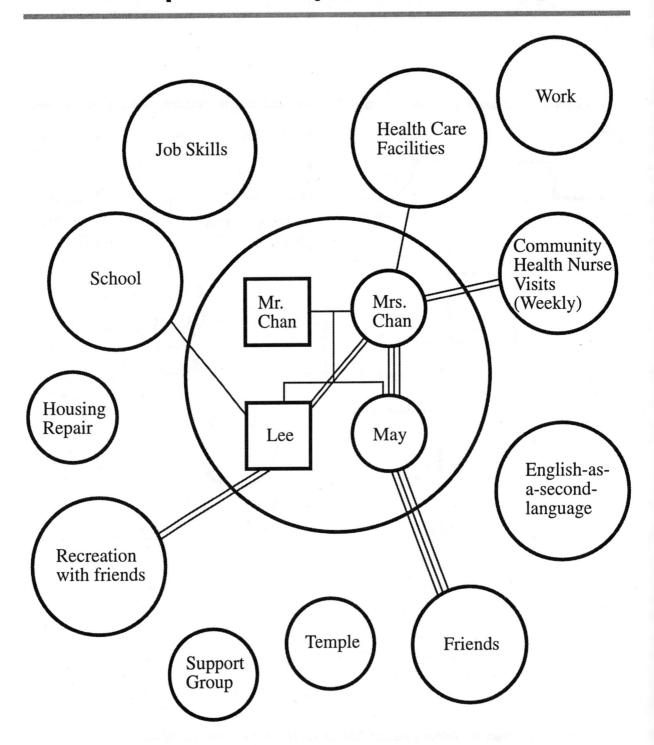

Figure 21-1
Wave Pattern of Violence

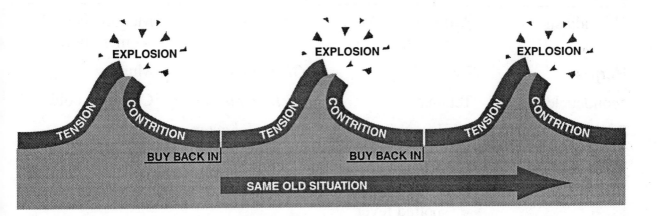

Redrawn based on cycle of violence from The Battered Woman by Lenore E. Walker. Copyright © 1979 by Lenore E. Walker. Reprinted by permission of Harper Collins Publishers.

Table 24–1
Examples of Types of Transmission for Various Communicable Diseases*

Direct	Indirect	‡Fecal-Oral	Airborne
Candidiasis	Arthropodborne viral diseases	Amebiasis	Meningococcal meningitis
Herpes	Lyme disease	*Giardiasis*	Mumps
Mononucleosis	Tetanus	*Escherichia coli*	Common cold
Syphilis	Onchocerciasis	*Campylobacter*	Rubella
Gonorrhea	Rabies	Hepatitis A	Pertussis
Ebola	Rocky Mountain spotted fever	Salmonellosis	Psittacosis
Cryptosporidiases	Diphtheria	Cholera	Influenza
Leprosy†	Taeniasis	Typhoid fever	Measles
Trachoma	Botulism		Tuberculosis
Viral warts	Dracunculiasis		Legionellosis
Chicken pox	Plague		
Yaws	Schistosomiasis		
	Yellow fever		
	Malaria		

*As communicable diseases, these diseases can occur in the individual, in the family, or in other aggregates or populations.

†Exact mode of transmission not clearly understood.

‡Transmission may be person-to-person or animal-to-person.

Table 24–2

Levels of Prevention of Communicable Diseases

Affected Population	Level		
	Primary	Secondary	Tertiary
Individual (AIDS)	Education Change sexual behavior/ other high-risk practices	Screening for AIDS in at-risk populations Reporting Early diagnosis and treatment	HIV drugs Maintain health Prevent conversion from HIV to AIDS Prepare for dying
Family (malaria)	Sleeping under bed net Protective clothing (long-sleeved shirts and long pants) Insect repellents Eliminate mosquito-breeding stagnant water/spraying of ponds	Reporting Immediate diagnosis and treatment of infected individuals	Prevent mosquito feeding on infected individuals Appropriate treatment using correct drugs to prevent further drug resistance
Aggregate (measles)	Education Measles vaccination Documentation	Screening for unimmunized individuals Early diagnosis and treatment Reporting Control of spread (epidemics)	Treatment of disease Epidemic measures

Table 26–3
Examples of Environmental Health Problems

Area	Problems
Living patterns	Drunk driving Involuntary smoking Noise exposure Urban crowding Technological hazards
Work risks	Occupational toxic poisoning Machine-operating hazards Sexual harassment Repetitive motion injuries Carcinogenic work sites
Atmospheric quality	Gaseous pollutants Greenhouse effect Destruction of the ozone layer Aerial spraying of herbicides and pesticides Acid rain
Water quality	Contamination of drinking supply by human waste Oil spills in the world's waterways Pesticide or herbicide infiltration of ground water Aquifer contamination by industrial pollutants Heavy metal poisoning of fish
Housing	Homelessness Rodent and insect infestation Poisoning from lead-based paint Sick building syndrome Unsafe neighborhoods

(Continued on next page)

Table 26–3, continued

Area	Problems
Food quality	Malnutrition Bacterial food poisoning Food adulteration Disrupted food chains by ecosystem destruction Carcinogenic chemical food additives
Waste control	Use of nonbiodegradable plastics Poorly designed solid waste dumps Inadequate sewage systems Transport and storage of hazardous waste Illegal industrial dumping
Radiation risks	Nuclear facility emissions Radioactive hazardous wastes Radon gas seepage in homes and schools Nuclear testing Excessive exposure to x-rays
Violence risks	Proliferation of handguns Increasing incidence of hate crimes Pervasive images of violence in the media High rates of homicide among young black males Violent acts against women and children

Table 27–2
Types of Occupational Hazards and Associated Health Effects

Category	Exposures	Health Effects
Chemical (routes of entry: inhalation, skin absorption, ingestion, and ocular absorption)	Solvents	Headache, central nervous system dysfunction
	Lead	Central nervous system disturbances
	Asbestos	Asbestosis
	Acids	Burns
	Glycol ethers	Reproductive effects
	Mercury	Ataxia
	Arsenic	Peripheral neuropathy
Biological (routes of entry: inhalation, skin contact or puncture, ingestion, and ocular absorption)	Blood or body fluids	Bacterial, fungal, viral infections Hepatitis B
Physical	Noise	Hearing loss
	Radiation	Reproductive effects, cancer
	Vibration	Raynaud's disease
	Heat	Heat exhaustion, heat stroke
Psychosocial	Stress Work-home balance	Anxiety reactions and a variety of physical symptoms
Ergonomics	Static or non-neural postures	Musculoskeletal disorders
	Repetitive or forceful exertions	Back injuries
	Lighting	Headache, eye strain
	Shift work	Sleep disorders
Safety	Electrical	Electrocution
	Slips and falls	Musculoskeletal conditions
	Struck by or against object	